When Violence

Erupts

A Survival Guide for Emergency Responders

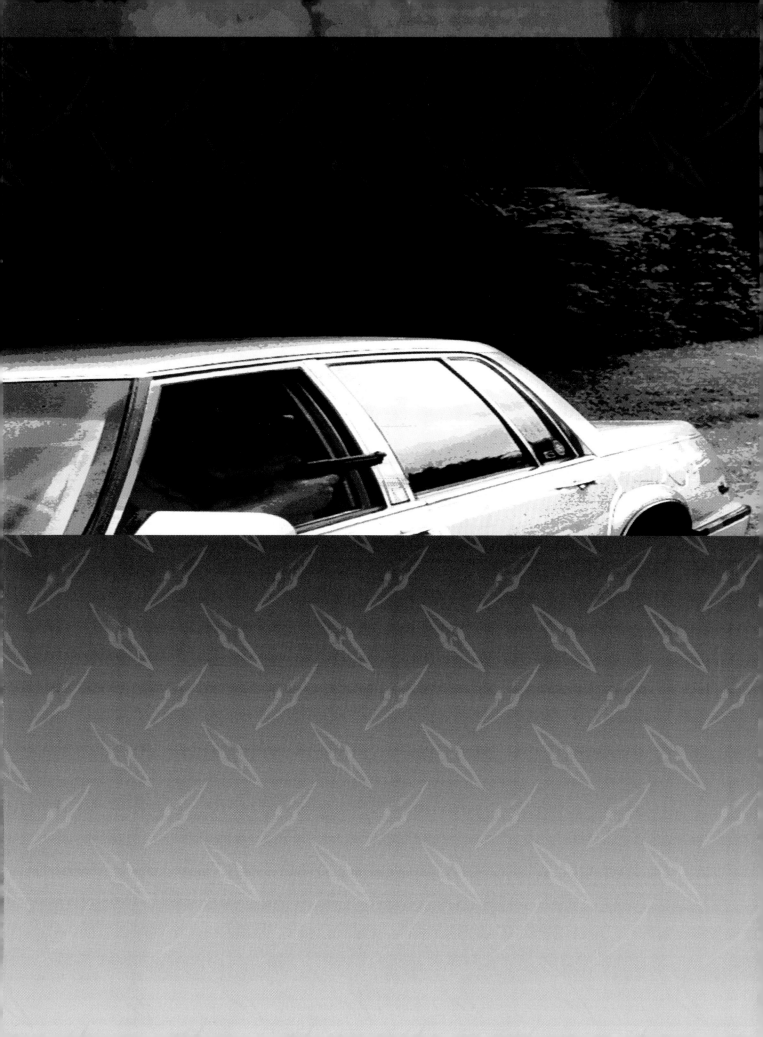

When Violence

Erupts

A Survival Guide for Emergency Responders

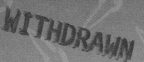

American Academy of Orthopaedic Surgeons

Author:

Dennis R. Krebs

Baltimore County Fire Department Baltimore County, MD

JONES AND BARTLETT PUBLISHERS

Sudbury, Massachusetts

BOSTON   TORONTO   LONDON   SINGAPORE

Library of Congress Cataloging-in-Publication Data

Krebs, Dennis R.
    When violence erupts: A survival guide for emergency responders / Dennis R. Krebs; American Academy of Orthopaedic Surgeons.
      p. cm.
    Includes index.
    ISBN 0-7637-2070-4
    1. Emergency medical personnel—Safety measures. 2. Emergency medical personnel—Crimes against—Prevention. I. Krebs, Dennis R. II. American Academy of Orthopaedic Surgeons. III. Title.

RC86.7 .K73 2002
362.I'8—dc21

2001058190

Printed in the United States of America
06 05 04 03 02   10 9 8 7 6 5 4 3 2 1

Contents

Chapter 1   The Threat and the Need 1

I Thought You Were a Cop! 3
I'm Not a Cop! 3
The Element of Surprise 4
Contrary to Previous Training 4

Chapter 2   Highway Incidents and Your Approach to the Scene . . . 6

Incidents That Indicate a Need for Caution 6
Positioning the Emergency Response Unit 7
Personal Preparations Before Leaving the Unit 8

Chapter 3   Approaching the Motor Vehicle 10

Driver-Side Approach 11
Passenger-Side Approach 15
Variation for Vans 17
The Head-On Approach 19
Time Frame for Starting Treatment 20

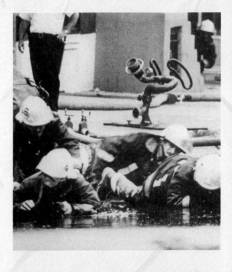

Chapter 4   Fleeing an Armed Encounter 22

The Armed Patient 23
Using the Vitals Pad as a Distraction Technique 26
Partner Down! 27
Backing Away from the Scene 28
Justifications for Backing Away 29
Calling for Assistance 30

Chapter 5   Residential Incidents 32

An Escalating Incident 33
Arriving on the Scene 35
Approaching the Residence 37

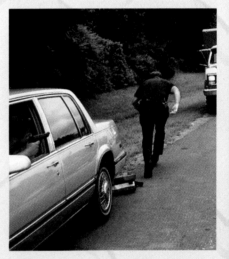

Chapter 6   Entering a Structure 40

Positioning at the Door 41
Moving Through the Entrance Way 42
Moving Within the Structure 43
Weapons in the Residence 44

Chapter 7   Domestic Encounters 46

Calm the Situation with Voice Control 47
Turn the Individual with Eye Contact 49
Body Language 49
Buttons 50
Tier System of Entry into an Unstable Area 50
Using Barriers to Separate Individuals 51
Distraction Techniques 51
Avoiding the Violent Situation 52

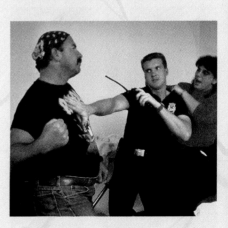

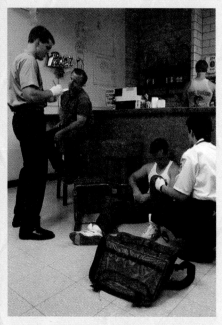

Chapter 8   Barroom Situations 54
Size Up 54
Entering the Establishment 55
Contact and Cover 56
The Hasty Retreat 56
Using Available Human Resources 57

Chapter 9   Cover and Concealment 59
Cover 60
Using Walls as Cover 61
Body Position 62
Changing Locations 62
Concealment 63

Chapter 10   Hostage Situations 64
Surviving as a Hostage 65
People Who Take Hostages 66
    Crazies 66
    Criminals 66
    Crusaders 66
Stages of a Hostage Situation 66
    Capture Stage 66
    Transport Stage 67
    Holding Stage 68
The Stockholm Syndrome 70
Law Enforcement Procedures in a Hostage Situation 70

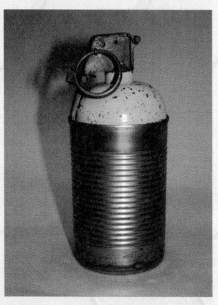

Chapter 11   Bombs, Booby Traps, and Makeshift Weapons 72
Who Uses Explosives? 73
Bombs and Explosives 74
Preparation and Preplanning 76
Reported or Suspected Bomb in the Area 77
Conducting the Search 79
Confirmed Explosive Device 79
Postexplosion Operations 80
Booby Traps 80
Makeshift Weapons 82

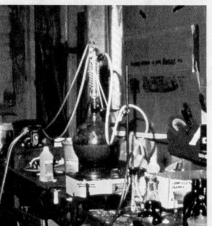

Chapter 12   Clandestine Drug Laboratories 90
Location of Illegal Drug Laboratories 91
Recognizing Illegal Drug Laboratories 91
Hazards Associated with Clandestine Drug Labs 93
Emergency Scene Operations 94
EMS Operations 95
Fire Suppression Operations 95
Positive-Pressure Ventilation 96
Monitoring Personnel Working in the Hot Zone 97
Interacting with a Methamphetamine User 97
Club Drugs 97
    Ecstasy 98
    LSD 98
    Date-Rape Drugs 99

Chapter 13   Self-Defense Tactics 101
Reasonable Use of Force 101
The Interview Stance 103
The Wrist Grasp 103
Technique for Distracting an Assailant 103
The Power of a Tweak 104
Breaking a Headlock 104
Breaking a Stranglehold When Attacked from the Front 104
Breaking a Stranglehold Applied from the Rear 105
Defending Against a Choke Hold from Behind 106
Breaking a Rear Bear Hug 106
Breaking a Stranglehold Applied from Above 107
Defending Yourself When Knocked to the Ground 107
Practice 107
Documentation 108

Chapter 14   Tactical Emergency Medical Support . . . 109
The Team 110
Goals of a TEMS Program 111
Training 112
Mission Planning 112

Chapter 15   Mass-Casualty Shootings 117
Preparation 117
Communications 120
Command 121
Operations 122

Chapter 16   Evidence Preservation 125
What Is Evidence? 125
Critical Issues at Violent Crime Scenes 126
Wound Ballistics 128
Clothing 129
Sexual Assaults 130
Critical Issues at Vehicular and Pedestrian Accidents 130
Documentation 130

Chapter 17   Gangs 133
What Is a Gang? 134
Gang Structure 135
  Territorial 134
  Corporate 134
  Scavenger 134
  Hardcore Members 134
  Fringe Members 134
  Wannabees 135
Specific Groups 135
  West Coast Gangs 135
  Midwest Gangs 135
  Hispanic Gangs 138
  Asian Gangs 139
  Motorcycle Gangs 140
  White Supremacist Groups 141
  Female Gang Members 143
  Gang Affiliations 143

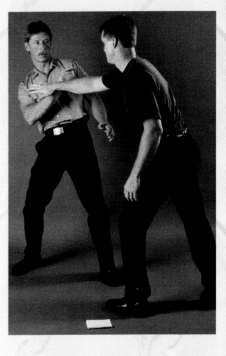

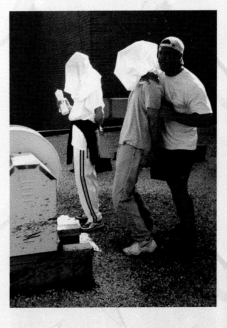

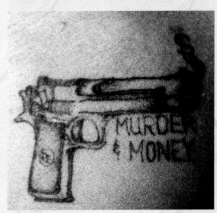

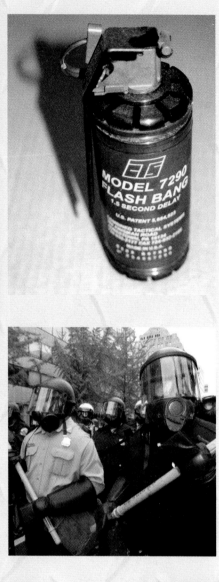

Graffiti. 144
Working in Gang Areas 145
Terminology 146

Chapter 18   Less Lethal Munitions 148
The Force Continuum 148
Tear Gas 149
OC Spray 151
Light/Sound Diversionary Devices 153
Tasers 153
Projectile Weapons 154

Chapter 19   Civil Disturbances 157
Planning 158
Strategy 161
Tactics 162
EMS Unit Tactics 164

Chapter 20   Patient Restraint 166
EMS Court Cases 167
Criteria for Restraint 168
Restraint Procedures 168
Recent Developments 169
Documentation 170

Chapter 21   Terrorism: Calibrating Risks and Response . . . 171
Overview 172
Biologic and Chemical Terrorism 173
Chemical Weapons 174
Military Chemical Agents 176
  Nerve Agents. 176
  Blister or Vesicant Agents 178
  Blood Agents or Cyanides 178
  Choking or Pulmonary Agents 178
  Irritants or Riot Control Agents 178
Biologic Weapons 178
  Anthrax. 180
  Botulinus Toxin 180
  Cholera 180
  Plague 184
  Q Fever 185
  Ricin 185
  Smallpox. 185
  Staphylococcal Enterotoxin B (SEB) 186
  Trichothecene Mycotoxins (T2) 186
  Tularemia 186
  Venezuelan Equine Encephalitis (VEE) 187
  Viral Hemorrhagic Fever (VHF) 187
  Summary 187

Appendix A   Incidents 189

Appendix B   Soft Body Armor 192

Notes 195

Index 203

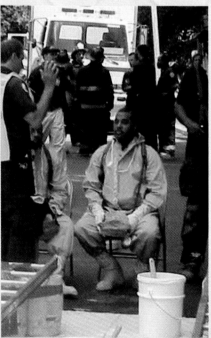

Acknowledgments

A number of individuals assisted in a variety of ways to allow this text to be published. My thanks to:

Colonel David B. Mitchell, Superintendent of the Maryland State Police and Trooper First Class Cynthia M. Brown of the Maryland State Police for providing personnel for photographs.

Jennifer Lofland, Intelligence Analyst with the Drug Enforcement Administration for providing information and photographs relating to club drugs.

Chief Terrence B. Sheridan of the Baltimore County Police Department and Lieutenant Kim Hall of the Forensic Services Section for supplying photographs for evidence preservation.

Chief William R. Bamattre of the Los Angeles City Fire Department for providing information and photographs from the 1992 civil disturbances.

Captain Patrick Shanley of Los Angeles City Fire Department Station 33 for graciously allowing the use of his personal photographs of the civil disturbances in 1992.

Walter Drivet of the Union County, New Jersey, Emergency Response Team for reviewing the chapter on "Mass-Casualty Shootings" and providing photographs.

Captain Richard Brooks III of the Baltimore County Fire Department for graciously providing his plane to take aerial photos and other classified missions (the secret is secure).

Mike Parlor of the Tactical Training Unit of the Los Angeles Police Department for information on Tasers.

Detective Teresa M. Krebs of the Baltimore County Police Department. She is my loyal supporter, cheerleader, best friend, and wife.

Reviewers

Sgt. Charles Angello
Essex County College Police Academy
Cedar Grove, NJ

James D. Davis
Ashburn, VA

Stephen J. Rahm NREMT-P
Department of Combat Medic Training
Boerne, TX

Gary Wiemokly
EMS Coordinator
St. Francis Hospital and Medical Center
Hartford, CT

Foreword

When I joined the Phoenix Fire Department and became a firefighter, I quickly learned that every time we operated in the street, there were lots of hazards present. In those (old) days, we did mostly fire fighting, so we always had to keep the fire from getting on us; stuff (like the building) would collapse on or under us, and it was really easy to get lost in the smoke and not make it back outside. As a young firefighter, I got beat up a lot (like most young firefighters), but tried to develop a set of survival skills so I could avoid those same painful experiences. When I became an officer, I attempted to develop the capability to manage my troops in a safe and survivable way. Throughout my career I have observed, studied, and thought about the physical hazards that affect the safety of firefighters. These physical hazards are the result of mostly physics, chemistry, engineering, and thermodynamics.

The development of EMS in our service has caused our personnel to personally interact and intensely "connect" with the people who receive our services in an entirely different way. While structural fire fighting includes mostly physical conditions, emergency medical services requires us to deal with human conditions. These situations can (and do) create highly emotional reactions in those who we meet at these incidents. Emotions like fear, anger, and pain can cause people to be violent and when our responders arrive to deliver service, that violence can be directed towards them. This violence has created a new set of hazards to our responders. Just like the old time physical hazards, we must keep from getting the violence on us. The situation can collapse on or around us, and we had better pay attention and be careful of where we go, because if we get in the wrong (unsafe) place, we won't make it back outside. Simply, violence can hurt us, trap us, and kill us just as quickly as the physical problems that we face on the fireground.

Dennis Krebs is a smart, experienced, modern guy who has done the same thing regarding how to survive the hazards created by violence that us old geezers did about structural fire fighting hazards. He has observed, studied, and thought about how we should conduct ourselves when violence occurs. He describes what happens in violent situations and how we can effectively react. He removes the mystery in a way that we can develop safe responses to situations that are just as predictable in human terms as the physical conditions are in burning buildings.

Pay attention as you read this book ... it could save your life.

Fire Chief Alan V. Brunacini
Phoenix Fire Department

Preface

While working a daylight tour of duty in early 1983, I was assigned to the medic unit operating out of the Towson Fire Station in Baltimore County, Maryland. The majority of the unit's first response district was a white-collar business community surrounded by quiet, upper-middle class residential areas.

Shortly after I assumed the duty, the dispatcher announced the first call for the tour: "Medic 1, respond to Charles Street and Kenilworth Drive for a possible heart attack; man reported slumped over the steering wheel." When the medic unit arrived on the scene, my partner and I found the driver slumped over the steering wheel in his car, which was stopped on the shoulder of the road. As we approached the driver's side of the vehicle, there was a strong odor of alcohol. Feeling that it was "just another drunk," I reached through the open window, touched the occupant on the shoulder, and told him to, "Wake up."

I was nearly killed when the subject sat up with a .357 Magnum in his hand and attempted to shoot me in the face. Fortunately a state trooper had approached the vehicle from the opposite side and was able to disarm the subject before anyone was harmed.

This incident represents the thousands of times each year that emergency responders face similar circumstances. Perhaps you found a single-shot pistol in the pocket of an accident victim complaining of neck and back pain. Or, maybe an intoxicated patient at a party tried to take a swing at your partner. After each such incident we simply wipe our brows and look up towards the heavens to give thanks. Perhaps, as you arrive home at the end of a shift, you give a tighter squeeze to your loved ones as they greet you at the door.

Increasingly, firefighters and emergency medical technicians are seriously injured and even killed in these violent confrontations. The six incidents listed below were denoted in the first edition of this text. Appendix A includes the numerous incidents that have occurred since the publication of the first edition of *When Violence Erupts*.

- Baltimore, Maryland Fire department medical personnel knocked on the front door of a house and were greeted by two arrows shot through the closed door.

- Bellevue, Tennessee Responding to a request for assistance, a firefighter was attacked and kidnapped. By the end of the incident the firefighter was dead.

- New Orleans, Louisiana Firefighters and police officers came under gunfire while extinguishing multiple fires set by a sniper/arsonist at a Howard Johnson hotel. Four emergency services personnel were killed and six were wounded.

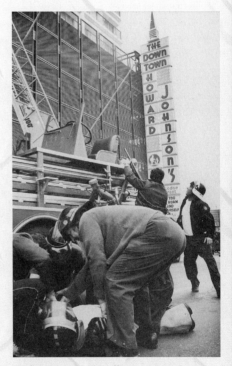

Firefighters and police officers came under gunfire while attempting to extinguish multiple fires set by a sniper/arsonist at a hotel. Four emergency services personnel were killed and six were wounded. *(Courtesy G.E. Arnold, The States- Item, Gretna, LA)*

- Pittsburgh, Pennsylvania   Paramedics were attacked and injured while attempting to provide medical assistance to the victim of a domestic disturbance. The assailant had objected to their giving care.
- San Ysidro, California   Engine crew members were pinned down by gunfire for 90 minutes during the McDonald's massacre.
- Philadelphia, Pennsylvania   Five firefighters were wounded when they were caught in a cross fire during a gun battle between police and the radical group MOVE.

Many emergency responders are surprised to hear that violence against our peers is so serious and widespread. Oftentimes they believe that these near-fatal incidents occur only in urban areas. Yet, the complacent attitude of personnel in suburban and rural areas leaves them open to the potential for serious injury. Many believe that "it can't happen here." Most certainly responders in Padukah, Kentucky, and Columbine, Colorado, had similar thoughts. Many of our own institutions, fire departments, rescue/EMS services, even state-wide EMS agencies have failed to identify this issue as a problem and support the needed policies, training, or publications that would improve the safety of our personnel.

To date there are still no national statistics on injuries to career and volunteer firefighters and prehospital care providers. However, a Chicago study showed that 96% of emergency medical technicians in major EMS agencies in cities across the United States had been assaulted in the line of duty (Walsh DW, Chicago, IL, master's thesis, 1993). This same study showed that 24% of the jurisdictions surveyed reported having personnel who had been shot and 80% of the jurisdictions had personnel who had been shot at. Chicago alone reported 180 assaults on ambulance personnel in 1 year.[1] New York City reported 161 assaults on their personnel in a similar time period.[2]

Defending yourself against violence is not part of your job. However, you need to know how to avoid violence when possible and how to protect yourself when it erupts. The purpose of this book is not to make you afraid to answer an alarm; it is to help you reach a middle ground where you can function both effectively and safely.

Since 1990 many fire departments and EMS services have used this text to train their personnel in avoiding violent confrontations. A number of law enforcement officials have also found this text useful. Without question firefighters and emergency medical technicians have returned home to their families at the end of a tour of duty due to the information contained in this text. I hope the new edition of *When Violence Erupts* will again cause each of you to hesitate ever so slightly when confronted with a potentially violent situation. Stay safe!

Dennis Krebs

Chapter 1

The Threat and the Need

Have you ever arrived at an incident only to find that the dispatcher's description did not reflect a true picture of on-scene conditions? This may not be the fault of the dispatcher. The dispatcher may not know that a person with "difficulty in breathing" was hit in the throat with a baseball bat. A caller who describes "severe lacerations" may really mean multiple razor cuts, and the "attempted suicide" victim may in fact have a gunshot wound in the back.

Whether you are responding to a call in a rural area, in a normally quiet neighborhood, or in the inner city, you should never be complacent about the possibility of encountering violence. Domestic fights; child, drug, and alcohol abuse, and similar problems occur at every social and economic level, in every type of community on a daily basis throughout our country. Each incident is a possible threat to the safety of emergency service providers who are untrained in personal protection tactics.

Many fire, rescue, and emergency medical service departments throughout the country are addressing the problem of violence in their communities in different ways, in part because it is becoming more difficult to ignore. Fire departments in Houston and the city of Los Angeles now provide paramedics with soft body armor for personal protection should they find themselves in a violent situation. In Branford, Connecticut, the local union purchased bulletproof vests for use by firefighters who respond to shooting or stabbing incidents.[1] Other agencies permit individuals who purchase their own soft body armor to wear it on duty.

Progressive departments are providing fire, rescue, and emergency medical personnel with basic training classes, continuing education seminars, and hands-on training in how to avoid violence and how to survive an incident that suddenly escalates beyond control.

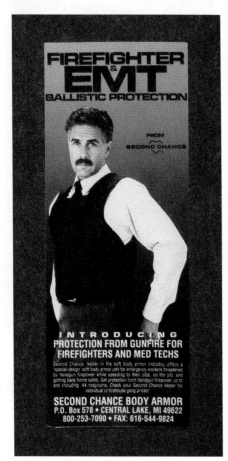

Figure 1-1 Brochure introducing ballistic protection for firefighters and emergency medical technicians that was distributed at the 1988 International Association of Fire Chiefs Conference. (*Courtesy Second Chance Body Armor, Inc., Central Lake, MI*)

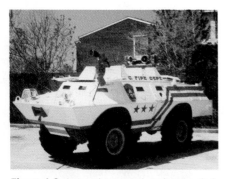

Figure 1-2 Armored personnel carrier operated by the District of Columbia Fire Department.

Individual emergency service workers throughout the nation confidentially admit to carrying small-caliber handguns, blackjacks, knives, or other weapons for self-protection without department authorization.

Companies selling personal protection products recognize the potential of the fire, rescue, and emergency medical services market for their products (**Figure 1-1**).[2] They advertise in professional periodicals and appear at association meetings and conventions. Fabricators of armor-plated vehicles advertise antiterrorist cabs for fire apparatus in fire service trade publications (**Figure 1-2**).[3]

A routine call may suddenly turn into a violent situation and cause further injury to the patient, injury to the rescuer, or even death. Without professional training, emergency service personnel must learn the hard way how to deal with situations that threaten their personal safety. But these experiences can result in serious injury to or the death of the emergency services worker (**Figure 1-3**). This book provides the basic tactics for personal survival and will help you recognize those situations that could be fatal if not handled properly. If you practice the techniques presented in this book on a daily basis, you should survive an unexpected eruption of violence.

The target audience for this book is every emergency services responder who arrives on the scene before law enforcement personnel. To develop the necessary survival techniques, these responders need realistic survival training similar to the training provided to law enforcement personnel. Because all emergency services agencies respond to potentially life-threatening situations daily, every responder should receive training in self protection. Self-defense techniques are important for anyone faced with an aggressive patient. Some situations will require you to use reasonable limits of force. Unfortunately, these skills are not taught in most emergency medical technician training programs.

Departments that encourage personnel to master survival techniques should experience a reduction in on-the-job injuries, long-term absences, and forced early retirements. If you are prepared to avoid or survive violence, you may experience less job-related stress and may be more able to handle assignments in high-risk locations.

The information in this text is not normally found in fire, rescue, or emergency medical services publications. This entire book is devoted to *your* survival. It is not information that should be shared with the general public. Your awareness of these survival tactics gives you the element of surprise; limited disclosure to others prevents the tactics from being used against you.

Although this information can help you avoid injury during violent incidents, situations can still go awry. You can follow every safety precaution and still be injured or killed while responding to an emergency. Many competent emergency services workers have died in the line of duty, even though they did everything right. Remember, if someone really wants to do you bodily harm, that person will find a way to accomplish the goal.

The threat is *there*, it is *real*, and it is *ever present*. The more you understand the threat of violence, the better your chances will be to avoid or survive a violent situation.

I Thought You Were a Cop!

Have you ever gone into a convenience store for coffee while on duty and received your coffee free because the clerk mistook your uniform for that of a police officer? Have you every been approached by a person from out of town who said, "Excuse me, officer, do you…?" This tourist also thought you were a police officer.

Many people mistake uniformed fire and rescue personnel for police officers. Compare the appearance of the two people in **Figure 1-4**. Both are wearing blue pants, white shirts, name tags, and breast badges. Both have patches visible on their sleeves. Both are holding flashlights and portable radios. Both have a bulge on their right hip. The difference is that the bulge on the police officer is a gun, and on the paramedic, it's a pouch with scissors, forceps, and other instruments.

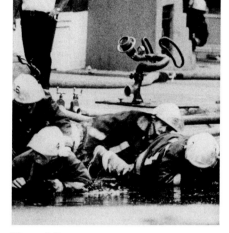

Figure 1-3 Firefighters scramble for safety when a gun battle breaks out between police and the radical group MOVE. *(Courtesy Wide World Photos, New York)*

In fireground situations, firefighters are wearing protective clothing, which readily distinguishes them from police officers. However, as the first responders to a medical emergency, firefighters may have their protective clothing in a side compartment of the medic unit or in the cab of the fire apparatus. Most fire departments consider it more professional to handle medical calls in clean uniform shirt and trousers rather than bunker gear.

The person whose consciousness has been altered by drugs or alcohol may confuse firefighters or medical personnel with law enforcement officers. The confusion created by the similarity in uniforms could result in a dangerous situation for the first responder.

For example, you arrive on the scene of a person slumped over the steering wheel. The medic unit has all warning lights operating, and the siren is still winding down as you get out of the unit. As you and your partner approach the vehicle, your attitude is, "I'm an EMT. I'm here to help this person." But the driver is remembering a judge's comment that if he is caught driving while intoxicated again, he'll be jailed. You are thinking, "I'm here to help," and he is thinking, "Here is a cop."

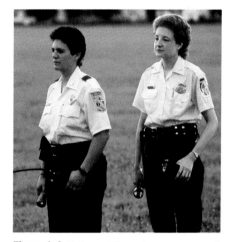

Figure 1-4 Uniformed fire and rescue personnel can be easily mistaken for police officers.

The driver saw the flashing lights; the fact that they are red and white and not red and blue made no difference. He heard a siren, saw the lights, and now he sees you standing there in uniform. He can't read the small print on the bottom of your patch that says **EMT** or **Fire Department.** Because of his recent trouble, all he sees is a police officer. In his condition he expects to see a cop, and so he does. He knows the cop would not be there to *help* him.

In this type of situation, you should anticipate that the individual may take some form of aggressive action. The action may be verbal abuse or a physical attack, with or without the use of a weapon.

To prevent cases of mistaken identity, some emergency response units have adopted a more casual uniform, with shirts that do not have badges, patches, or collar devices. Only the department logo is printed on the left breast pocket. Other departments have authorized crew neck pullover t-shirts with the department's initials over the left breast and on the back of the shirt.

I'm Not a Cop!

The nonchalant attitude of many firefighters and emergency medical technicians as they approach an unknown situation places their personal safety in jeopardy. Someone may be waiting to give them an attitude adjustment in the form of a gun in the face or a knife in the back.

When a call comes in for a shooting, stabbing, domestic assault, severe lacerations caused by a fight, or similar incident, law enforcement personnel are usually dispatched at the same time as fire and rescue units. However, fire and rescue personnel may arrive on the scene before law enforcement personnel.

In rural areas, there may be more volunteer fire or rescue service workers than law enforcement personnel for an entire jurisdiction. In urban areas, police assistance may not be available during peak trouble hours.

Until recently, most personal survival training programs have been directed toward the law enforcement community. This has caused a problem for fire, rescue, and emergency medical services personnel who arrive at a dangerous situation while law enforcement personnel are still en route to the scene.

The Element of Surprise

Most fire and rescue personnel do not have the authority to carry firearms, nor do they have the power to arrest someone. Therefore, it is important to maintain an *element of surprise* to offset this disadvantage. Many tactics and techniques not known by the general public are available to emergency services workers. The public will not expect you to take such actions. People who see you approach a motor vehicle or a building will not know that you are analyzing and measuring the situation against a series of systematic checks in your mind. This element of surprise is the major form of self-protection available to fire and rescue personnel—its importance cannot be overemphasized.

Contrary to Previous Training

The fundamental principle in every first responder and emergency medical technician training program has been, and in most cases still is, patient care. Stopping to think, "Hey, slow down, what about my safety?" is not emphasized. As a result, fire and rescue services personnel fully realize the importance of handling trauma or treating the medical emergencies, but downplay concerns about personal safety.

Until recently this thinking permeated the entire emergency services field. Hazardous materials training now advises that rescue personnel no longer rush right into the scene. Tactics courses now teach the importance of slowing down: stop and check the nature of a vehicle's contents, do not enter what appears to be an unsound structure, and do not attempt body recovery until the cause of death is known.

Should your response to a potentially violent situation receive the same cautious treatment as your response to a hazardous material situation? Yes! When you respond to a call involving a gunshot wound, you may think MAST trousers (Military Antishock Trousers), IVs, and helicopter transport. You should also be thinking, "Where is the person who pulled the trigger? Is the scene secure? Is the area safe to enter?" If you are shot on arrival, you are no help to the patient or to your partner.

The degree of caution used during responses to fire and hazardous materials emergencies has increased markedly over the past 15 years. Responses to medical emergencies should also include a degree of caution. You should not charge through the door of a residence to aid a shooting or stabbing victim without law enforcement assistance. You should not remain in an area where verbal abuse could lead to physical abuse. Sometimes you may be in the middle of administering assistance when violence erupts. If this happens, you must leave the dangerous and violent situation. The victim you leave behind may die—you will not.

When trouble occurs, you may not have time to load and package the victim on a backboard in the proper manner. However, you may be able to grab the victim by the ankles and run. The victim may incur some additional injuries, but sometimes you will have little choice. Ask yourself, "Do I stay and continue to treat the patient while risking the possibility of being injured or killed myself, or do I leave the area immediately and, if time allows, drag the patient too?" Your first concern is to look out for yourself.

SURVIVAL TIPS

1 Even if you sincerely believe that your primary concern must always be for the patient and that these ideas are too radical, please do not stop reading.

2 This book will introduce you to ideas that can alter your attitude and help you stay alive to treat another patient on another day.

3 First responders in large cities are aware of increasing personal danger. Responders from suburbia may not expect sudden violence. Just because it has never happened to you does not mean it will not happen on your next call.

4 Unless your department has trained you to use a weapon and officially authorizes this practice, *do not* carry small-caliber handguns, blackjacks, knives, or other weapons for self-protection.

5 Possession of an unauthorized weapon may result in legal and civil liabilities for you. A weapon may give you a false sense of security and be used against you.

6 You must recognize the possibility of violence developing on every call.

7 NFPA 1500, *Fire Department Occupational Safety and Health Program,* requires your organization to provide you with training that will ensure your ability to perform your assigned duties safely.

Highway Incidents and Your Approach to the Scene

Interstate highways were built to move goods and products necessary to maintain our standard of living, military personnel and equipment in time of a national emergency, and the motoring public. Regretfully, our highways are also used to transport illegal drugs, weapons, and other contraband, as well as criminals and undocumented workers.

The problems occurring on interstate highways may also be found on intrastate highways, city streets, narrow rural roads, and parking lots. Emergency responders must be aware of the potential danger on any call involving a motor vehicle, regardless of the location. The danger may range from minor physical abuse from an intoxicated driver to potential death if illegal drugs are being transported.

Incidents That Indicate a Need for Caution

Traffic accidents, including those involving personal injury, usually are not dangerous situations for emergency services personnel who arrive to render assistance. However, many incidents should feel uncomfortable to you and indicate that you should exercise caution as you approach the stopped vehicle. Examples of these incidents include:

- Even though your emergency vehicle siren is going and the maximum number of warning lights that the electrical system can support are operating, there is no movement or sound coming from the stopped vehicle. Heads are visible, but no one turns around. This is not the normal response to your arrival. If someone in the vehicle requires assistance and if someone in the vehicle is awake and responsive, the normal reaction would be for the alert, responsive person to turn and look in your direction. If everyone in the vehicle continues to sit facing forward without moving, your suspicions should be heightened.

- You arrive on the scene of a reported cardiac arrest that occurred in a vehicle. You find the vehicle correctly parked on the side of the right-of-way with no visible occupants. This, too, is an abnormal situation. People seldom pull off to the side of the road, put their vehicle in park, lie down on the seat, and die. Usually, the vehicle is found stopped at an angle, against the guard rail, or in the ditch.

- You stop your unit to the rear of a vehicle reported to contain an injured person. Suddenly everyone gets out of the vehicle and starts walking toward your unit. Could one of them be injured? Who called for assistance?

- The driver of the vehicle adjusts the rearview or side mirror as you exit the unit and watches your every move.

- The vehicle and the occupants appear out of place for the neighborhood. Could the crossing of invisible ethnic boundaries have caused the existing situation? Could the situation escalate?

- Visible signs of violence such as guns, knives, or other weapons are lying in the street. Where are the people who used them? Do they have other weapons?

- You must enter a dimly lighted area or an area with limited exit (escape) routes such as a deserted highway, a dark country road, or an inner-city alley. Constantly maintain a sense of caution when you are in precarious situations.

- You have a "gut feeling" that something is not right as you approach the scene. Do not ignore this feeling. Analyze the cause before you proceed.

As your level of concern increases, you should decide on a firm course of action. Either continue to respond as you normally would and walk up to the vehicle, or call for law enforcement assistance and wait until the scene is declared safe.

If you request law enforcement assistance each time you enter a questionable situation however, you may soon develop a reputation for *crying wolf*. This action is not conducive to a good relationship with the law enforcement community or a sign of professionalism. However, if you are trained to carry out the systematic approach procedures described in this chapter, it will not be necessary to call for law enforcement assistance in most incidents. These procedures should be used every time you believe impending danger exists.

Positioning the Emergency Response Unit

Whenever feasible, approach stopped vehicles from the rear. Exceptions to this rule will be discussed in Chapter 3. The unit should be positioned a minimum of 15' to the rear of the stopped vehicle on a

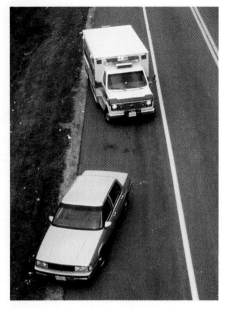

Figure 2-1 Position the unit a minimum of 15' to the rear of the stopped vehicle on a 10° angle to the left.

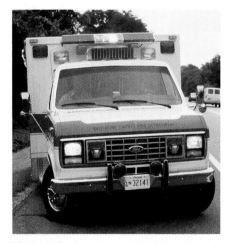

Figure 2-2 If gunfire erupts from the stopped vehicle before you pass the frontal plane of the response unit, the turned wheels provide a protective area for you.

10° angle to the driver's side (**Figure 2-1**). As you bring the unit to a stop, turn the wheels all the way to the left. In this position the engine block of most units and the wheels of all units can be used as protective areas should violence erupt.[1]

The density of the engine block and the wheels will stop a bullet fired from a .357 Magnum, but a .22 caliber bullet may penetrate the door area of the unit. If an occupant exits a stopped vehicle and begins shooting at you, the engine block and the wheel areas offer you the most protection (**Figure 2-2**).

Always position your unit in a way that provides you with maximum protection. An improperly positioned unit can be a disadvantage to the responder who must approach a stopped vehicle, especially during the night.

Personal Preparations Before Leaving the Unit

When you arrive at the scene, do not leap out of your unit, grab the jump kit, and run up to the vehicle. Before leaving the unit, allow yourself several moments to inspect the scene for safety.

As the driver positions the unit, the person in the right front seat should record the license plate number of the stopped vehicle. Include the name of the state where the license tag was issued. Before you leave the unit, place this information in a predetermined location, such as next to the radio (**Figure 2-3**). Now, if something happens to you and your partner, a written record of the vehicle exists. The advisability of giving this information to the communications dispatcher has been discussed with people working in communications centers throughout the country. Their consensus is that dispatchers may disregard the information as unimportant because they do not routinely receive this type of information. Writing the information down and placing it by the radio before you leave your unit is in your own best interest.

When incidents occur after dark, the unit driver should use the high-beam headlight setting to illuminate the interior and the perimeter of the stopped vehicle. In units equipped with a spotlight, the driver can shine the spotlight into the rearview mirror of the vehicle (**Figure 2-4**).

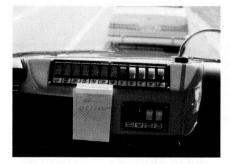

Figure 2-3 Before you leave the unit, write down the license number and state of the stopped vehicle and place the information in a predetermined location.

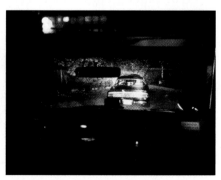

Figure 2-4 A normal medic unit light package will illuminate the interior and perimeter of the vehicle.

This will usually illuminate the interior of the passenger compartment. Emergency vehicles not equipped with spotlights may carry hand-held quartz lights, which the driver can aim at the rearview mirror of the vehicle. A properly aimed spotlight or quartz light will prevent the occupants from seeing the responder approach the rear of the vehicle.

When the emergency response unit is properly positioned, you can approach the driver's side of the vehicle without casting a shadow in the side or rearview mirrors (**Figure 2-5**). Even though the unit lights are shining on your back, the 10° angle of your unit to the vehicle means that your shadow will fall in the roadway instead of on the vehicle's mirrors. Do not walk between the spotlight and the vehicle. Doing so will momentarily provide a silhouette in the vehicle's rearview mirror and alert the occupants to your exact position. Strategic use of lighting is essential to the element of surprise.

Each rescuer should take a flashlight when leaving the unit, but the light should remain off until the approach is complete and there is a need to see inside the vehicle.

When leaving the unit, always remember to carry a pad of paper to record vital signs and other pertinent patient information. Many rescuers carry a small pad of paper in their shirt pocket whenever on duty. Carry the pad in your left hand when making all of the approaches discussed in Chapter 3. Using the pad as a distraction technique will be discussed in Chapter 4.

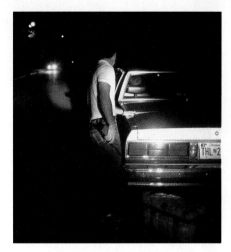

Figure 2-5 When the unit is properly positioned, your shadow will be cast in the roadway rather than in the vehicle's mirrors.

SURVIVAL TIPS

1. Most vehicles are equipped with a door-activated switch that automatically turns on the interior lights when a door is opened. Disconnect this switch to prevent lighting the interior of the unit. After you determine that the scene is safe, you can activate the interior light with the manual dash switch.

2. Notice whether the occupants of a vehicle you are approaching at night adjust their mirrors to prevent your lights from reflecting inside of their vehicle. This is a potentially dangerous situation. Request law enforcement to investigate. Withdraw the rescue unit to a safe area and wait until the police arrive.

Chapter 3

Approaching the Motor Vehicle

Many law enforcement personnel who die in the line of duty each year receive the fatal wound after leaving the relative safety of the patrol car to approach a stopped vehicle. Because of this, law enforcement agencies have devised and refined various techniques that allow personnel to approach a stopped vehicle safely.

In recent years, these techniques have been assembled into an approach system that emergency medical service responders can also use. When it is used properly, this mental checklist provides a maximum degree of safety.

An approach system is not usually needed on incidents such as personal injury accidents at a busy intersection, accidents where the vehicle is found torn wide open, or situations with bystanders already around the vehicle. These calls are obvious; you have been thoroughly trained to handle these situations, and they present a minimal amount of danger to your personal safety.

An approach system is most beneficial when you sense something on arrival that gives you a very uncomfortable feeling about approaching the vehicle. This simple and systematic procedure can be easily adapted for use by all emergency services personnel.

After you have properly positioned your emergency response unit and have completed all the necessary preparations before leaving the vehicle (see Chapter 2), you may begin your approach. When there are two or more responders in the unit, the person riding in the right front seat of the emergency vehicle makes the approach. This person is usually the officer in charge (OIC) of the emergency vehicle and the most experienced member of the crew.

Many law enforcement agencies use two officers when approaching a stopped vehicle (**Figure 3-1**). If one of the advancing officers is attacked, the other officer can use deadly force if necessary to neutralize the situation. Firefighting and emergency medical service agencies are not equipped with the necessary weapons or authorization to respond in the same way. A single-person approach procedure exposes only one person to a possibly dangerous situation. All other members of the emergency response team remain with the medical unit or engine company in case something goes wrong.

Driver-Side Approach

Anyone who has been stopped for a moving violation knows that the law enforcement officer usually walks up the driver's side of the vehicle to the window and asks for a driver's license and registration. This approach is so common and has been used by law enforcement personnel for so many years that the driver is often holding the license and registration out the window by the time the officer reaches the side of the car.

Although this approach seems very straightforward, there is in fact a systematic method that the officer uses in moving from the patrol car to the side of the stopped vehicle. Law enforcement officers use this method so automatically that the general public does not even recognize it. All emergency services personnel should become proficient in making this approach because of the protection it affords.

The approach begins when you, as the OIC, get out of the right side of the rescue vehicle. Close the door quietly to maintain the element of surprise. If you slam the door, the occupants of the vehicle will know by the noise that you have left the unit. With the door closed, the driver will be able to move the unit quickly, if necessary. Remove only the jump kit (aid bag) from the unit for the initial approach.

Do not take the electrocardiogram (ECG) monitor, oxygen, or other gear to the scene unless there is an obvious emergency. An excessive amount of equipment may interfere with your ability to move quickly. At this time you are the *only* person to leave the unit and approach the vehicle. Until you determine that the scene is safe, all other personnel should remain in the unit.

After you leave the rescue vehicle, walk around the rear of the vehicle and continue walking forward on the driver's side. Stop at the driver's door (**Figure 3-2**). Because the situation could change while you are behind the rescue unit, move around the rear of the unit as quickly as possible. If you arrive on the scene alone, start the approach from the driver-side door. You do not have to pass around the rear of the unit.

If you are assigned to a busy company, you may not always feel like walking all the way around the unit. In fact, you may not feel like doing any more walking than is absolutely necessary. But no matter how tired you may be, make it a habit to walk behind your unit instead of walking between the two vehicles. The extra steps could save your life. Some examples of why you should not walk between the vehicles include the following:

- If you walk between the two vehicles at night, you will be silhouetted by the headlights of your own unit. The occupants of the vehicle will know exactly where you are, and you will lose the element of surprise.

- If your vehicle is struck from behind, you may be crushed between your unit and the stopped vehicle.

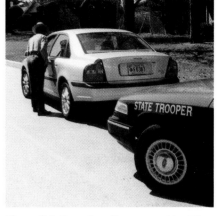

Figure 3-1 The police officer approaching this automobile is prepared to use force to control the situation.

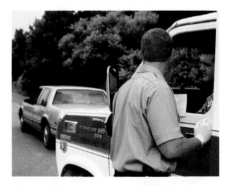

Figure 3-2 Before approaching the stopped vehicle, the officer in charge walks around the unit and stops at the unit driver's door.

- While you are between the vehicles, the driver of the stopped vehicle may accidentally shift into reverse instead of park, which may make the vehicle lurch backward.
- The person in the other vehicle may be wanted by the police. The driver may intentionally shift into reverse to injure you and gain time to escape in the ensuing confusion.
- If either vehicle accidentally rolls toward the other, you may be crushed between them.

When you reach the unit's driver-side door, discuss any changes in the overall situation with your driver. The emergency vehicle driver's responsibility is to observe the occupants of the vehicle in front while you walk around the unit. If either you or the driver notice any signs of danger, stop the approach and request law enforcement assistance. Danger signals include the driver's positioning the mirror to view your approach or heads popping up from the back seat and then disappearing. If you decide to abort the approach, the unit's driver should back the unit a safe distance away from the other vehicle and call for help. Until law enforcement personnel arrive and declare the vehicle safe, all emergency services personnel should remain in a protected area (**Figure 3-3**).

If you continue the approach, you will enter the open area between the front of your unit and the rear of the car. You have very little protection in this area. Make this portion of the approach quietly and quickly. Lift your feet when you walk; do not kick the gravel. Try to prevent keys or pocket change from jingling.

Move directly from the left front fender of your unit to the rear driver-side trunk area of the vehicle. Quietly put the jump kit on the ground near the back of the vehicle's trunk. Place the jump kit where you will not trip over it if you need to make a hurried retreat. Place your right hand lightly on the seam between the trunk lid and the left quarter panel (**Figure 3-4**) and check for any evidence that the trunk lid is not secure. Hand placement should be light enough not to move the vehicle. If the trunk lid feels abnormally higher than the left quarter panel, the lid may not be latched and someone may be hiding in the trunk. If the lid is ajar or if you feel movement in the trunk, slam the lid to prevent the occupant from exiting the trunk. Do *not* lift the trunk lid to close it—simply push it down instead. If you lift the lid and then slam it, you lose the element of surprise. You let the occupants of the vehicle know exactly where you are and that you are suspicious of the situation. If this happens, your life is in danger and you are no longer in control of the situation.

Avoid the area near the trunk lock. An armed occupant in a trunk may fire through the vehicle and try to hit anyone thought to be preparing to insert a key in the lock.

A "click" may indicate that someone has unlocked the trunk from inside the vehicle. If you hear this sound, immediately abort the approach and retreat to a safe location. To learn to recognize this sound, stand near the rear of a vehicle while a friend unlocks the trunk from inside the vehicle.

In the fall of 1972, officers from the Montgomery County Police Department in Maryland arrested the only apparent occupant of a vehi-

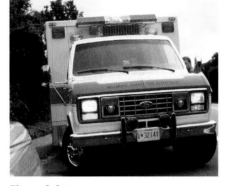

Figure 3-3 The OIC is protected by the front left fender and front left wheel, which can stop a .357 Magnum. When crouched close to the floor, the driver is protected by the engine block.

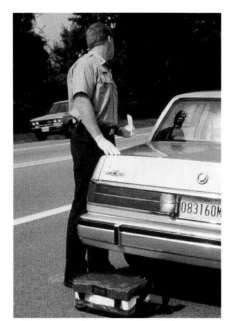

Figure 3-4 If the situation gets out of control and your life is endangered, do not stop to pick up the jump kit.

cle. He and another man were wanted for the armed robbery of a local shoe store. The car was impounded and towed to the Silver Spring Police Station for processing. During the investigation, officers found it difficult to gain access to the trunk of the vehicle. A police lieutenant attempted to enter the trunk through the back seat. He was shot in the forehead by the second robber who was hidden in the trunk (Gabriele M, Baltimore, MD, personal communication with Ludington G, 1988). If you do not develop and follow a systematic procedure that includes checking the trunk lid, you may be emergency medical technician or firefighter who is killed or wounded in a similar situation.

After ensuring that the trunk lid is secure, observe the side-view mirror. If the mirror is moving or appears to be at a strange angle, ask yourself, "Why?" If you are satisfied with the answer, move forward on the driver's side of the vehicle until you reach the "C" column (**Figure 3-5**). Moving belly-in toward the vehicle creates as small an image as possible for the occupants of the vehicle to see and keeps you out of the flow of traffic. Anyone who has worked a highway incident knows that some motorists do not slow down for any reason. If you are standing away from the side of the vehicle, you may be hit by passing traffic.

Some irresponsible truck drivers play a game called "dusting a trooper." Spotting a trooper standing next to a stopped vehicle, the truck driver maneuvers the truck as close as possible to the side of the road and tries to make air rushing from the side of the passing tractor-trailer blow the trooper's hat off. Just because you are not a trooper does not mean that this could not happen to you.

Always stand sideways to the vehicle and stay as close to the vehicle as possible. You will then have maximum protection from the occupants of the vehicle and from irresponsible motorists that pass.

Stop at the left "C" column and look in the rear and side windows (**Figure 3-6**). Notice the number of people in the vehicle. Pay particular attention to the location of their hands. Try to see what items are lying on the seat or on the floor. Look for weapons. If you see a high-threat weapon such as a gun or knife (**Figure 3-7**), abort the approach, retreat

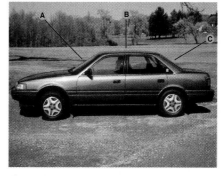

Figure 3-5 "A," "B," and "C" columns of a vehicle.

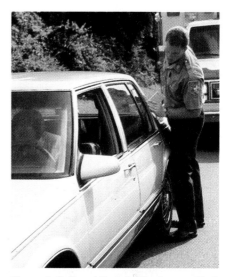

Figure 3-6 Stop at the left "C" column and look in the rear and side windows. Until the OIC declares the vehicle safe, the jump kit remains on the ground at the rear of the vehicle.

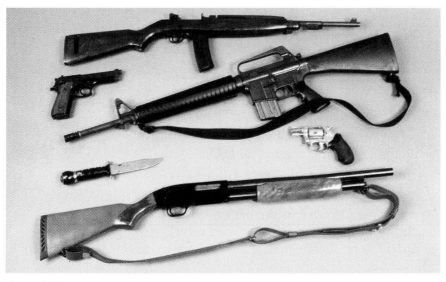

Figure 3-7 The primary purpose of high-threat weapons is to kill.

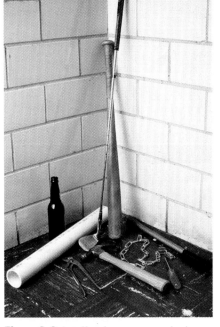

Figure 3-8 Low-threat weapons can also be used to kill; however, this is not their primary purpose.

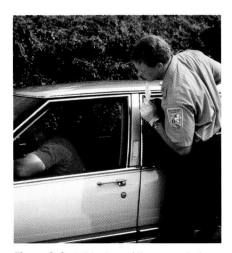

Figure 3-9 At this stage of the approach, do *not* move past the "B" column for any reason!

to a protected area, and call for police assistance. Once you abort the approach, do not resume the approach until law enforcement personnel arrive on the scene and declare the vehicle safe.

The presence of low-threat weapons should heighten your awareness of potential danger. Anything that can be used as a weapon but is not in the high-threat weapon category is considered a low-threat weapon (**Figure 3-8**). Innumerable items normally found inside a vehicle can be considered low-threat weapons, including things like a tire iron, a jack handle, a beer bottle, or a flashlight. You can do nothing about these items, but you need to be aware of their presence in case one of the occupants makes a sudden move toward the object. Unless there is an indication that the occupants of the vehicle intend to use the weapons against you, do not abort the approach. If a move is made, recognize the unexpected threat and immediately retreat to a protected area. The procedures for an aborted approach are the same, whether the danger is from low-threat or high-threat weapons.

If the back seat is occupied, do not pass the "C" column. If you pass the "C" column, the back-seat passengers will be behind you. You will have to divide your attention between the front and rear seats, which places you in an unfavorable position. When working an incident, treat rear-seat passengers and anyone standing behind you as potential threats. Exercise caution any time a civilian is standing behind you.

If there are no passengers in the back seat or any visible high-threat weapons, move forward to the "B" column with the same belly-in movement. As with the "C" column, the "B" column will conceal you from the passengers of the vehicle. Before attempting aggressive action, a driver posing a threat would have to turn in the seat, see you, and focus on you. As long as you remain behind the "B" column, you should have time to retreat to a safe area. Do *not* proceed to the driver's door at this time (**Figure 3-9**). Instead, run down a mental checklist about the front seat situation. Ask yourself, "Where are the occupants' hands? What are the occupants doing? Are any weapons visible?"

The front-seat area of a vehicle contains many places to conceal a weapon. These locations include the following:

- On top of the sun visor
- Under either side of the seat
- In the glove box
- In side-door pockets
- In the center console
- Between bucket seats
- Next to the driver's right thigh
- In the dashboard (**Figure 3-10 A-B**)
- In the steering wheel (**Figure 3-11 A-B**)

Be especially alert to the possibility of a gun next to the driver's right thigh. Because the driver is the person usually in charge of a civilian vehicle, anyone approaching a stopped vehicle is expected to walk to the driver's door. If you approach the vehicle as expected, you will not see a weapon next to the driver's thigh. Watch the occupants' hands; their direction of movement may give away the location of an unseen weapon. The innocent-looking model car attached to the dashboard speaker grill in **Figure 3-10 A** and **B** could also be a handle to remove the grill for quick access to the two semiautomatic weapons and extra ammunition concealed under the grill.

When you are ready to let the driver know that you are there, do so without moving past the "B" column into the driver's door area. Law enforcement personnel refer to this area as the *kill zone*. Dangerous situations in this area include the following:

- The driver can push the door open and knock you off-balance. If this happens, you have lost control of the situation and your life is in danger.

- A .22-caliber bullet is capable of passing through a car door. If a handgun is lying on the driver's lap, all the person has to do is pull the trigger when you reach the driver's door. Then you become part of the problem.

- If you pass the "C" column with the back seat occupied, you face the same threats.

Tap lightly on the window of the vehicle to get the driver's attention and announce yourself: "Pikesville Fire Company, do you need assistance?" There can be no doubt that you are from the fire department or ambulance service. Make it clear that you are there to help the patient. You do not want to be mistaken for a police officer.

Do not reach inside the car for any reason. The driver can grab your arm and pull you into the car or against the roof. This situation may result in your injury or death. You will be safer if you conduct the primary survey while you are concealed by the "B" column. Once you determine that the driver needs medical care, check that the vehicle is in park, and signal for the medic unit driver to move forward with the additional equipment.

After the OIC declares that the incident scene is safe and determines that the occupants of the vehicle need medical or other assistance, all personnel on the scene should follow the standard operating procedures for their department.

Passenger-Side Approach

Approaching the vehicle from the passenger side enhances your element of surprise and therefore increases your odds of survival if violence erupts.

After you complete the necessary preparations in the unit (see Chapter 2), begin your approach to the vehicle. The OIC is again responsible for making the approach but, in this example, the approach will be along the passenger side of the vehicle.

The occupants of the vehicle will expect you to approach the driver's side of the vehicle. The driver will usually be looking in the side mirror for you to make the usual approach, and the occupants will be waiting for you. If you systematically approach the vehicle from the passenger side, the occupants of the vehicle will be surprised when they see you, and you may be surprised at what you see.

A Maryland State Police trooper made a night stop of a vehicle and carried out all of the systematic checks during the approach from the

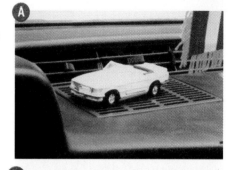
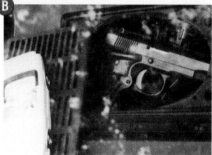

Figure 3-10 Dashboard hazards. **A.** Grill in place. **B.** Grill removed. *(Courtesy Colin Perkins, Bath Police Department, Akron, OH)*

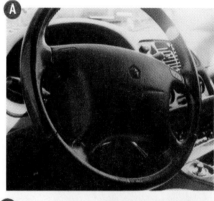
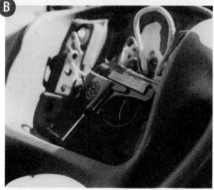

Figure 3-11 Steering wheel dangers. **A.** All new vehicles have driver and passenger supplemental restraint systems. **B.** With the airbag removed, it becomes the perfect place to conceal a small caliber handgun.

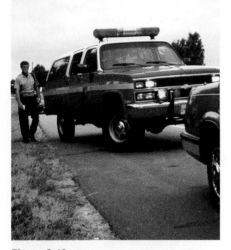

Figure 3-12 The passenger-side approach requires the person who has responded alone to exit from the driver's door and walk around the rear of the unit.

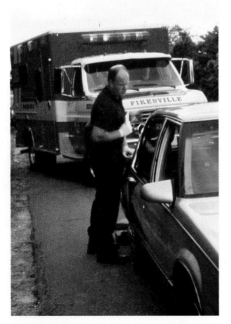

Figure 3-13 The officer in charge moves from the right front of the unit directly to the right rear-trunk area of the vehicle.

passenger side. As the driver watched the side mirror for the approaching trooper, the officer stood by the right "B" column and saw the driver stuff bags of marijuana under the front seat (Gabriele M, personal communication with Beard RJ, 1989). When the trooper tapped on the right-side window, the driver turned with an "I'm caught" look and started removing the bags from under the seat. If the approach had been from the driver's side of the vehicle, the trooper would not have seen this movement; it could have been a weapon instead of bags being concealed.

In single-person response units, the driver must exit from the driver's door and walk around the rear of the unit as the OIC did in the first approach discussed (**Figure 3-12**). In response units with more than one person, you (the OIC) exit from the passenger door with the jump kit and proceed quickly and quietly to the trunk on the passenger side. Ensure that your unit is properly parked on a 10° angle with the wheels cut to the left (see Chapter 2). Remember, as soon as you step out of the unit you are completely exposed. There is no protection from the unit as in the driver's side approach. Do not hesitate after exiting the unit. Proceed directly to the rear passenger-side trunk area and place the jump kit at the rear of the vehicle out of the path of travel (**Figure 3-13**).

Check the trunk lid to ensure that it is properly closed. Remember to use only a light touch on the trunk seam to detect motion or an unsecured trunk lid.

Using the same belly-in movement, proceed to the "C" column on the passenger side of the vehicle. Make the same checks for high- and low-threat weapons, and observe the occupants of the back seat. What are they doing? Where are their hands?

After you find that the back seat is safe, continue to the "B" column. Keep your belly in toward the vehicle. Check for high- and low-threat weapons. How many people are in the front seat? Where are their hands? While you check the front-seat area, use the "B" column for concealment and protection.

Stay out of the kill zone. Remember that the person in the passenger seat can give you the same problems as the driver who is being approached on the driver's side. If you are standing in the kill zone, both the passenger and the driver have a straight shot at you when they turn to acknowledge your presence.

Recognize that most weapons will be hidden with the expectation that the approach will be on the driver's side of the vehicle. When you are standing on the passenger side, you are in the best possible position to observe any device that could be aggressively used against you, but you must stay behind the "B" column.

After determining that the vehicle and the occupants are not a threat, announce your presence in a similar manner as described for the driver-side approach. Complete the scene size-up and notify your partner that it is safe to approach the vehicle. Your partner can bring any additional equipment that may be needed.

Law enforcement agencies, emergency medical services, and fire departments that use both the driver-side approach and the passenger-side approach claim that a greater margin of safety is available to personnel that use the passenger-side approach. The reasons stated include:

- You are out of the flow of traffic.
- A greater variety of cover is available.
- The distance between the driver and the emergency medical technician is greater; allowing the emergency medical technician more time to react to an aggressive movement.
- The interior design of most vehicles does not allow for quick movements to the right. For example, the driver cannot point a gun at a person standing behind the "B" column without moving over the seats or the headrest.

It is best to use the driver-side approach during daylight. The occupants of the stopped vehicle can watch you through the rearview mirrors regardless of the side of approach. The passenger-side approach has the greatest advantage during low-light conditions and at night with heavy shadows and strong lights providing protection.

Be prepared for the occupant(s) to be uncomfortable with your approach on the passenger-side. The driver may ask, "What are you doing over there?" or insist that you, "Come around to this side!" Your response should be, "Well, sir (or ma'am), I would prefer to work from this side. Please open the passenger-side door for me." If this happens, you will know that your approach from the passenger side has put the occupant(s) off-balance. Use this information to your advantage. Take control of the situation. Let the occupant(s) know, in a professional manner, that you are in charge. Remain on the passenger side.

Variation for Vans

Historically, van stops have been the most dangerous traffic stop for law enforcement officers. A van may be occupied by a single person driving or contain as many as 15 people that cannot be seen (**Figure 3-14**). Vans can carry many types of cargo, and the inability to see that cargo is a danger to responders. During a gasoline shortage, an Ohio man installed a 275-gallon fuel tank in his van to transport stolen gasoline (**Figure 3-15**). Consider the hazards that a vehicle like this presents if it is involved in a traffic accident.

Vans have been used to transport arms used by both motorcycle gangs and terrorist groups. Often when a motorcycle gang is riding in formation, at least one van is usually close behind, carrying the gang's weapons. Large-caliber machine guns mounted for firing out of the rear doors are also a possibility.

When approaching a van, exercise extreme caution. Because there are too many doors to watch simultaneously, the opportunity for one or more passengers to exit and come up behind you is a danger.

The driver-side approach is not recommended when approaching a van. Since you would be approaching the van from the opposite side of the sliding door, you would think that it would be the safer side. It is not — the occupant(s) will be expecting you to approach this side and will be able to anticipate your position.

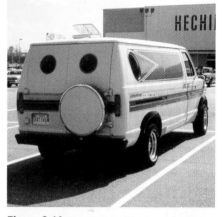

Figure 3-14 Vans are capable of carrying large numbers of people, contraband, and hazardous cargo.

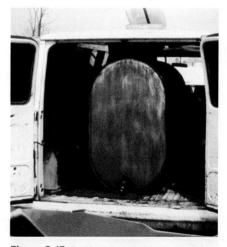

Figure 3-15 Fuel tank installed to transport gasoline illegally. (*Courtesy William Ennis Sr., West Carrollton Division of Fire, West Carrollton, OH*)

When using the driver-side approach on a van, you do not have the element of surprise because there is no "C" column to pause behind as you check the rear of the vehicle for weapons and occupants. Because of the way that vans are built, your first contact with the occupants will be when you reach the "B" column. Even then, you will probably be unable to see the front seat area from this position due to the height of the door window. You cannot see a passenger in the right front seat without stepping in front of the "B" column and placing yourself in the kill zone.

For example, a Maryland State Police sergeant stopped a van on the eastern shore of Maryland. The van matched the description of one thought to be carrying armed robbery suspects. The sergeant positioned the cruiser at the "B" column of the van and was talking door-to-door with the van driver. An unseen occupant sitting behind the driver placed a shotgun against the inside of the sheet-metal van, pulled the trigger, and killed the sergeant. The passenger who did the shooting did not have to see the target. The killer knew exactly where the trooper was stopped.

All approaches to vans should be made from the passenger side. Preparations for the approach are the same as described in Chapter 2. As part of the preparation and before leaving the unit, you and the unit driver should carefully look at the rear doors of the van. Agree on the condition of the doors (latched, unlatched), and on an audible warning signal that the unit driver will sound if the position of the rear doors or the driver's door changes during the approach. You will not be able to check the rear doors as you would a trunk lid when you approach the van.

The actual approach is a modified version of the passenger-side approach. When approaching a van, do not move forward on the side of the van or use the belly-in method recommended for the other approaches. If you are belly-in to the van, an occupant may suddenly open the side door and grab you. Instead, you will keep your distance.

In van incidents, you may get your shoes dirty. When you exit the unit with the jump kit, move 10' to 15' away from the passenger side of the van. If you have to jump a guard rail or walk in a ditch, do so. Remain clear of the side door of the van throughout the approach (**Figure 3-16**). From this distance, walk parallel to the van until you are approximately 45° forward of the "A" column.

The position shown in **Figure 3-17** gives you the greatest visibility inside of the van but keeps you at a safe distance until you can determine that the situation is secure. The occupants are not going to expect you to be in this position. By maintaining the element of surprise, you effectively control the situation.

From this point, you can announce your presence. Identify yourself as "Fire Department" or "Emergency Medical Services" and ask, "Did you call for an ambulance?" If you are satisfied with the answers and can see that medical assistance is required, call for the rest of the crew to meet you at the van and begin treating the occupants according to your standard operating procedures.

If there is no response to your calls, no one visible from your position, and no indications that this is other than a normal incident, move quietly to the "A" column and look on the floor of the van. The patient may be lying there in cardiac arrest.

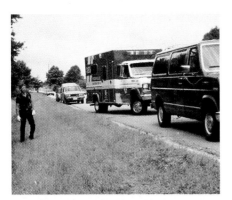

Figure 3-16 Until you are 45° forward of the "A" column, maintain 10' to 15' between yourself and the passenger side of the van.

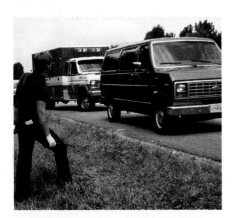

Figure 3-17 Position yourself 45° forward of the "A" column before making contact with the occupants of a van.

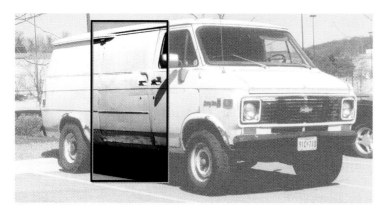

Figure 3-18 The area near the side door is known as the *grab area*. Attempting to flee past this area increases your chance of being injured.

If aggressive action from the van's occupants causes you to flee from your position near the "A" column, you may have to seek cover away from your emergency response unit (see Chapter 9). Do not run directly to the emergency response unit if you are in a position near the front of the van. If you do, you will pass near the side door of the van, which increases your chances of being attacked (**Figure 3-18**).

Foggy or tinted windows can obscure your view inside a vehicle. If the vehicle has foggy or tinted windows, approach it using the variation for vans. Usually the windshield is clearer than the other windows and you will be able to scan the interior of the vehicle.

The Head-On Approach

In some circumstances, positioning the emergency response unit at the rear of the vehicle in question is not practical; for example, you may be approaching the scene from the opposite direction of travel or the vehicle may be located in a parking lot (**Figure 3-19**). If you continue past the vehicle to turn around and approach from the rear, you lose the element of surprise. In these situations, use the head-on approach.

This approach requires the emergency response driver to stop the unit approximately 15' from the front of the vehicle on a 10° angle to the unit driver's left. If the call is a night response, place headlights on high-beam and aim any spotlights through the vehicle's windshield to conceal your exit from the unit. Follow all other preparations for leaving the unit described in Chapter 2.

Exit the unit with the jump kit, walk around the rear of the unit, and stop at the driver's door for updated information on activity in or around the vehicle. After determining the safety of the approach, move away from the passenger side of the vehicle for a distance of 10' to 15'. Walk parallel to the vehicle until you reach a position approximately 45° behind the vehicle. From this position move directly to the right rear trunk section of the vehicle, place the jump kit on the ground, and proceed with a normal passenger-side approach (**Figure 3-20**).

This modified passenger-side approach is recommended for day and night responses that require a head-on arrival at the scene. The rescuer using this approach can remain clear of the kill zone while attempting to reach the recommended position at the "B" column of the vehicle.

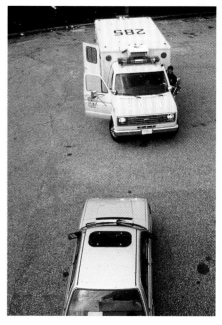

Figure 3-19 Not all approaches are made to the rear.

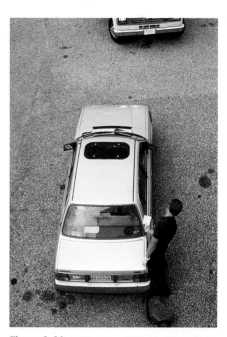

Figure 3-20 Until you are 45° behind the vehicle, maintain 10' to 15' between yourself and the passenger side of the vehicle. Once you reach this position, proceed with a normal passenger-side approach.

Time Frame for Starting Treatment

When you arrive at the scene, pause momentarily to assess your surroundings before you start treating the patient. After ensuring your personal safety, you can make a systematic approach to the vehicle in a timely manner, recognize the occupant's problem(s), and initiate basic and advanced life support consistent with accepted practices.

You may be questioned by your superiors, the press, the victim, or the victim's relatives or attorneys about why you took these precautions before starting treatment. Your best defense is that you were making sure the scene was safe for you to get to the vehicle and assist the patient without putting yourself in jeopardy. The Department of Transportation (DOT) *National Standard Curriculum for Emergency Medical Technician— Basic National Standard Curriculum* requires a check for scene safety.

The methods of approach described in this chapter do not take a great deal of time to complete. With proper training and practice, you should be able to complete the approach and begin treatment within 30 to 45 seconds after you leave the unit.

SURVIVAL TIPS

1) Some incidents obviously require the presence of a law enforcement unit before you approach the vehicle, such as when people are holding weapons or yelling and cursing at you. Other situations are not so obvious. No hard-and-fast rules define what is a go or no-go situation. If you feel (for whatever reason) that you may be in danger, *do not approach the vehicle.*

2) Your license or contract does not require you to place yourself in danger of bodily harm just because you are wearing an emergency medical technician or fire department patch. If you are uncomfortable with a situation, you can use the public address system on your unit to give instructions to the occupants of the vehicle before you leave the unit.

3) Directing occupants of a vehicle to turn on their interior light before you start a night approach will enhance your ability to identify how many occupants are in the vehicle, where they are in the vehicle, and any potentially hostile movements they may make during your approach (**Figure 3-21**). Illuminating

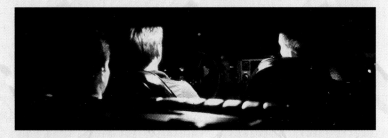

Figure 3-21 Before starting a night approach, direct the occupants of the vehicle to turn on the interior light.

the interior light may also help conceal you from the vehicle's occupants.

4 If you are alone in responding to an incident, take a portable radio with you when you leave the unit because no one else will be able to call for assistance if something happens. Make sure the portable radio is on low volume before you exit the unit. You do not want to lose the element of surprise because of an unexpected radio transmission from another unit on the same frequency.

5 Flashlights should remain off until needed. Hold the light at arms-length and away from your body before you turn it on (**Figure 3-22**). Illuminate the scene for only a few seconds during each use.

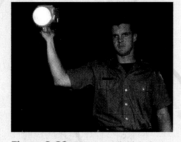

Figure 3-22 Because a light makes a good target, hold a flashlight away from your body when illuminating an area.

6 If all four doors of the vehicle open and all of the occupants start walking toward the emergency response unit, use the public address system. Tell them to return to their vehicle. The scene is easier to control when the occupants remain inside of the vehicle rather than wandering around outside. If they ignore your instructions, you are still in a position to back away from the scene (see Chapter 4).

7 If you are in a single-person response unit, you can create the effect of more than one rescuer during a night approach by slamming the door of the unit twice. Reinforce this illusion by carrying on a conversation with your imaginary partner who remains unseen on the other side of the vehicle. If the unit is properly positioned (see Chapter 2), your headlights or spot light will prevent the occupants of the vehicle from seeing you approach.

8 Do not become complacent—repetitive calls with no problems can have a deadly effect. Consider the need for using an approach system on each incident involving a motor vehicle.

9 Vehicles operated by high-ranking government officials, heads of large corporations, or your local drug dealer may be equipped with heavy armaments or armor plating. Optional equipment on these vehicles may include smoke grenade or tear-gas launchers located behind the front and rear bumpers or in the trunk compartment.[1]

4

Fleeing an Armed Encounter

A systematic approach to a stopped vehicle provides you with some degree of safety. However, you still don't know what you will find in the vehicle. The driver or occupants may be armed; they may be running scared or they may have a calculated plan to entrap you. They may be faking an injury, or there may be a real emergency. Imagine yourself in the following scenario:

You are dispatched to a car stopped on the side of the highway. The dispatcher described the situation as a "man having difficulty breathing in a motor vehicle." You make a systematic approach along the driver-side of the vehicle. When you reach the "B" column, you announce yourself, "Woodlawn Fire Company, are you okay?" The driver turns in the seat, and you see a pistol in his right hand. What would you do?

If you are confronted by someone with a loaded gun, you need to know what steps you can take immediately to save your life. All people have an instinctual "flight or fight" response to danger. But this response must be controlled to be effective. Fortunately, an occupant seated in a motor vehicle must make several moves to initiate aggressive action against a rescuer who is properly positioned to the rear of the appropriate column. For example, an aggressor armed with a gun must:

- **TURN**—Physically turn in the seat, so that the trunk is twisted toward the rescuer
- **LOCATE**—Visually locate the rescuer
- **FOCUS**—Focus on the rescuer to accurately take aim
- **FIRE**—Point and fire the weapon

Each of these actions takes time. You need to know how to make the best possible use of this time to successfully avoid the intended aggression. If you can interrupt any of these steps, you increase your chances of surviving a shooting incident.

Statistics published by the Federal Bureau of Investigation (FBI) show that most shootings are not like those depicted in television programs.[1] They do not occur at 100 yards, nor do they involve innumerable rounds of fire. A shooting is a very intimate experience. Usually the participants are less than 5' apart, and the incident is generally over in less than 4 seconds, with a total of three rounds fired.[2] Your survival may depend on any action that delays the aggressor from firing, and increases the time you have to escape. The techniques outlined in this chapter are designed to give you that extra bit of time.

The Armed Patient

In addition to knowing how to respond to an actual threat, you should also know what to do in case of a potential threat. For example, you are called to the scene of a personal-injury accident. You find a single vehicle that has crashed into a tree. The lone occupant of the vehicle is a male, approximately 35 years old. He appears to be awake, but he is slow to respond. Because yours is the only unit on the scene, you systematically approach the vehicle, determine it is a legitimate incident, and signal your partner to join you. You announce, "Fire Department Paramedic, we're here to help you. Where do you hurt?" The driver responds with several moans and some movement of the arms and upper body. As you complete the scene size-up, your partner opens the driver's door, and the first thing you both notice is a 2" revolver stuck in the patient's belt. He has no holster, just the pistol (**Figure 4-1**).

At this point, you should stop and ask yourself, "Who is this guy?" He is probably not a law enforcement officer because a police officer seldom carries a gun without a holster. It is an unsafe practice—the gun may go off. Also, most law enforcement officers purchase their own off-duty weapons. Because they want a weapon they can rely on, they take care of it. A holster prevents the gun from falling on the ground, keeps the gun clean, and keeps the gun oil from soiling clothes. Seeing a gun without a holster should alert you that the person is not authorized to have a gun, and is possibly carrying the gun illegally.

In a situation where the gun is in a holster or if you have a gut feeling that the individual may be a police officer, ask, "Are you on the job? What agency are you with?"

In any case, you must make a decision. Do you attempt to take the gun? Do you back off and call for the police? Do you ignore the gun and continue to treat the patient? Or do you send your partner to summon the police while you treat the patient? Your decision also depends on whether you are alone and on how badly the patient is injured.

In this example, the patient is in no immediate danger. He has a good airway and no severe bleeding. You have time to consider several options. With the patient's altered mental status, he may be too dangerous to treat safely as long as he has the weapon. Before continuing treatment, you would be well within the limits of acceptable patient care to back off to a safe distance and call for law enforcement personnel to take the gun, particularly if you are alone.

If you elect to continue treatment without waiting for law enforcement assistance, attempt to gather more information about the patient. Position yourself where you can see the gun as you ask the patient about his iden-

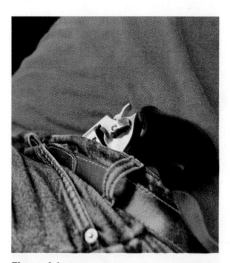

Figure 4-1 Because most law enforcement officers do not carry a gun unless it is in a holster, finding a gun in this position indicates a need for caution.

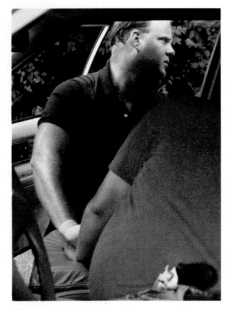

Figure 4-2 "I need to check your pulse and blood pressure."

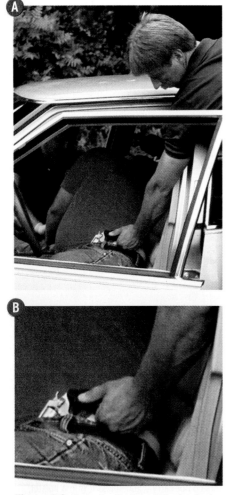

Figure 4-3 Disarming the immobilized patient.

tification, medical-assistance cards, and allergies. Check his wallet for identification. If you find a badge, ask the patient what agency employs him. Do not ask leading questions such as "Are you a cop?" because they would probably result in an affirmative answer. Because you cannot be sure that the patient is telling you the truth, tell him that you feel uncomfortable because he is armed but do not attempt to take the gun. Based on extensive training, law enforcement officers will not surrender a weapon that may be used against them. Even though the patient is lethargic, do not attempt to remove the gun. A struggle may result, and the gun may accidentally discharge. Attempting to grab the weapon exposes you, your partner, and your patient to unnecessary danger.

If the patient is unconscious or shows no signs of aggression and you decide to proceed with treatment, immediately take the patient's radial pulse. Take the pulse on both wrists at the same time, and continue to take it until the patient is disarmed (**Figure 4-2**). As you perform this procedure, you can subtly immobilize the patient's hands against the steering wheel, which should allow your partner to disarm the patient safely (**Figure 4-3 A-B**).

In some situations, you may not be able to wait until law enforcement personnel arrive on the scene to assist in disarming the nonaggressive patient. Because of various factors, 20 minutes or more may pass before the first police officer arrives. The courts may consider this an unnecessary delay in starting treatment. You should take into account your past experiences and familiarity with local law enforcement, traffic and weather conditions, location, and proximity to assistance, as well as the patient's condition and response when deciding whether to attempt to disarm a patient.

If you notice a weapon in the vehicle but not physically on the person, consider moving the person away from the weapon rather than attempting to move the weapon away from the person. During a frontal impact, objects on or under the seat may be thrown forward onto the floor. If you see a weapon on the floor between or near the patient's feet, leave it there. When you touch or pick up the weapon, you become part of the chain of custody and may have to testify in court if illegal weapons or other unlawful contents are found in the vehicle.

Never leave the patient alone if you can see a weapon in the vehicle. Send someone else to get the additional equipment you need from your unit. If the patient is conscious and oriented, you can use extrication as an excuse to immobilize the patient's hands. As you apply the cervical collar and the short backboard (or Kendrix Extrication Device [KED] if available), explain that you must immobilize the patient's hands and that you will release them as soon as the transfer to the medic unit is complete. At the same time, you or your partner should secure the patient's hands together with gauze dressing. Once the patient is clear of the vehicle, assign someone from the response team to secure the vehicle until law enforcement personnel arrive and accept custody of the vehicle and its contents.

If you must take custody of a gun, write down the make and model and lock the weapon in the drug box, drug cabinet, glove box, or another secure location until you can turn it over to law enforcement personnel. *Never* place the weapon on the roof of the vehicle, the street, or the other end of the bench seat in the car. Do not stuff the gun into your own waist belt or back pocket. When law enforcement personnel arrive on the scene, locate the officer who is responsible for writing up the incident. Write down the name, identification or badge number of the officer, and the case number assigned to the incident before turning over custody of the weapon. Document all of this information on your run sheet, including where you found the weapon. If the patient is a law enforcement officer, treat the officer's badge with the same degree of importance as you treat the gun.

Often, weapons are not carried in the open but are hidden on the person. When you conduct a scene size-up and an initial assessment, you can check for weapons while you check for injuries. As you run your thumbs around the inside of a patient's belt to check the pelvis, spinal column, and abdominal rigidity, you may find handguns, knives, or other weapons. Do not neglect the extremities—leg and ankle holsters are very popular. If you find one weapon, look for more. Be alert for weapons that do not look like weapons: for example, a derringer attached to a belt buckle or a pen that is actually a pistol (**Figure 4-4**). Additional information on makeshift and concealed weapons is in Chapter 11.

There are subtle clues that may indicate that a person is carrying a weapon. However, you must be observant to pick up on these clues. When arriving at an emergency, you are taught to observe the scene. At a fire emergency, you look for the color and density of smoke. At a medical call, you look at the patient's general appearance to form an initial impression. You will use these same skills to identify someone who might be armed.

Detective Robert Gallagher of the New York City Police Department examined over 1,000 arrests that were made by fellow officers.[3] He wanted to know if a person carrying an illegal weapon exhibited any changes in normal body language. They do. However, unless emergency medical responders are trained to recognize this type of behavior, they will miss these cues.

There are two issues that provide a base for identifying someone who might be carrying an illegal weapon. First, most criminals do not carry their firearms in a holster. Second, as with the rest of society, most criminals are right-handed. By keeping these two facts in mind we can begin to predict where people carry guns. Many criminals carry their weapon in either a right-front pocket or right-rear pocket. Another location will be in the waistband of their pants—either near the small of their back or behind their right hip. Since it "looks so cool on the cop shows," some criminals will have the gun stuffed down their waistband just

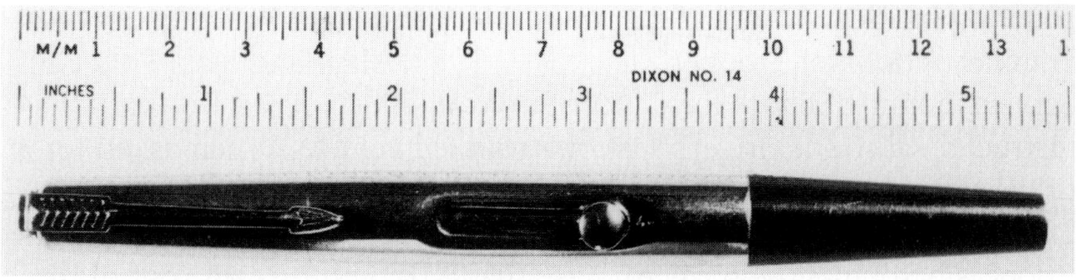

Figure 4-4 Many weapons do not look like weapons. This pen fires a small-caliber round. (*Courtesy Baltimore City Police Department, Baltimore, MD*)

in front of their left hip. This allows for a rather impressive "cross draw" where the criminal reaches across his or her body to grab the concealed gun.

People who do carry a gun in their right-front pants pocket may keep their right hand in that pocket so that the outline of the gun will not be visible. If the gun is being carried in a pant's waistband, a hand in the right pocket is often needed to prevent the gun from falling through the waistband and dropping onto the ground. Since the weight of the gun will tend to pull the pants down, the person may be continually tugging up on his or her pants. The person will also continually check to see that the gun is still in place either by placing his or her hand on the weapon or by pressing his or her arm against the side of his or her body. When the person walks, you might observe one foot dragging slightly and the natural swing of the arms may be abnormal on that same side.

Is the person's clothing abnormal for the season? A heavy coat worn in warm weather may conceal some type of weapon—possibly a shotgun. If it is extremely cold and his or her jacket is not zipped or buttoned closed, it may be open to allow quick access to some type of firearm. Does the coat hang lower on one side or swing abnormally when the person turns? Is the collar tight against the back of the neck or one side? For instance, if the collar of a coat is tight against the left side of a person's neck, he or she may be carrying a gun in the right-side pocket of the jacket. Is the person wearing only one glove in cold weather, keeping the other ungloved hand in a coat pocket? His or her other hand, usually the right, may be caressing a semiautomatic pistol (Hobson RA, Collins CE, Metropolitan Police Department, Washington, DC, *Identifying Characteristics of the Armed Gunman*, unpublished document, 1995).

If you pick up a patient from a police station or jail, never assume that a complete search has been made. As a provider of prehospital care, you must conduct a survey of your patient. Use the opportunity to search for weapons. Be careful because razor blades and other small, sharp objects may be hidden in cuffs, in the lining of a jacket, pants, or hat, and even in hair.

Using the Vitals Pad as a Distraction Technique

Distraction techniques are very useful in breaking the chain of events (turn, locate, focus, and fire) in a shooting incident. Again, the purpose of the distraction is to increase your chances of survival by giving you time to escape. The distraction does not have to be elaborate, as this story shows.

While conducting drills at the Maryland State Police Glen Burnie Barracks, Trooper First Class (TFC) Raymond J. Beard taught a technique that successfully disrupted the chain of events in an intended shooting incident 12 out of 12 times (Maryland State Police In-Service Training School for Trooper First Class, 1983. Maryland State Police In-Service Training School for Officer Survival, 1987). A state police instructor sat in the driver's seat of a stopped vehicle. When asked for a driver's license, the instructor drew a weapon and squeezed the trigger in a simulation of shooting the approaching trooper. TFC Beard told the troopers participating in the exercise that if something came out of the vehicle at them, they were to take off their Stetson[4] with their left hand (driver-side approach) and throw it at the eyes of the person behind the wheel of the stopped vehicle. The intent of this action was to make the armed person blink or flinch. Throwing the hat was 100% effective—in each case the person with the weapon either misfired or misaimed.

When something is coming at you, your initial instinct is to blink or flinch. Consider what happens when you are driving during a heavy rain and a passing vehicle throws water on your car's windshield. Even though you know the water is not going to hit you, you still blink or flinch when the water strikes the windshield. This is the reaction you want to provoke in your assailant.

Throwing your vitals pad at the person provides the same distraction as the water hitting the windshield or the troopers throwing their hats. It interrupts the chain of events long enough to permit you to get out of the line of fire and run to safety.

Carry the pad in your left hand when you make a driver-side approach. When in position behind the "B" column, raise the pad to your left shoulder. If the vehicle's occupant takes aggressive action during your initial interview, be prepared to throw the pad directly at the aggressor's nose (**Figures 4-5** and **4-6**). Use only a soft pad of paper for this technique. A hard object such as an aluminum report book or clipboard may cause needless injuries to the occupant of the vehicle. The soft pad will not cause undue harm. If the person is reaching for a lighter instead of a weapon and you react by throwing the vitals pad, you only have to apologize and explain. Exaggerate if necessary; say you just returned from a call where the patient took aggressive action toward you, and you thought it was going to happen again.

After you throw the pad, do not wait for a reaction. As soon as it is out of your hand, turn to your right (toward the unit), get out of the possible line of fire, and run to safety. Do not stop and pick up the jump kit—*run!*

The object is to put as much distance as possible between you and the aggressor. If possible, run to the unit (**Figure 4-7**). You can call for help or drive to a safer location. If you are cut off from the unit, evaluate the surrounding area for the best possible cover and concealment (see Chapter 9).

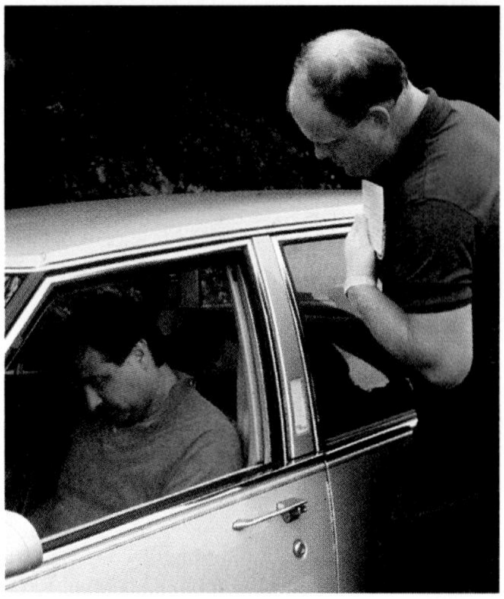

Partner Down!

As a member of an emergency response team, you rely on your partner every day. The experiences you've shared with each other create strong bonds. Imagine how you would feel if you saw your partner suddenly turn from the approach with a look of panic and start to run toward the unit. What would you do if, after several steps, your partner falls face down in the dirt with a bullet in the back?

Your initial reaction might be to get out of the unit and run to your partner. But that is potentially the worst action you can take in such a situation. If you leave the unit, you put both you and your partner in a dangerous and unprotected position. Plus, there is now no one in the unit who can call for assistance.

The proper action is to shift into reverse and step on the accelerator. Backing away from your partner may be the toughest decision you will

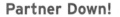

Figure 4-5 When conducting the initial interview, hold the vitals pad in the left hand and raise it to the left shoulder.

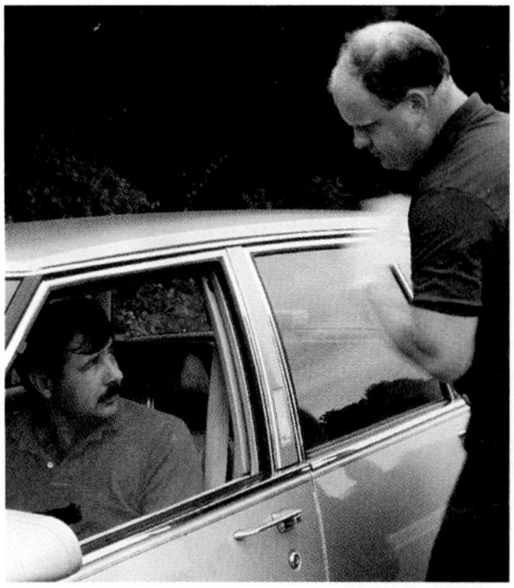

Figure 4-6 If aggressive action occurs, throw the pad directly at the nose of the aggressor.

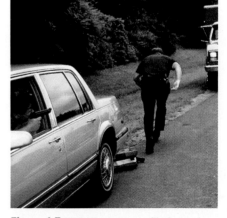

Figure 4-7 While the aggressor flinches and attempts to refocus, run toward the unit.

ever have to make. But doing so may give you the time you need to call for help.

When you make that call, do not scream into the microphone and then run to help your partner. Stay calm, stay on the line, and provide the dispatcher with all the information you can. If you get out of the unit, you will probably get hurt, and both you and your partner will lie there bleeding until help arrives.

You can probably think of several offensive actions that you would prefer to take, instead of backing away from your partner. These might include:

- Ramming the aggressor's vehicle
- Running down the aggressor with the unit
- Placing the unit between the aggressor and your partner

Any of these suggestions may be successful in a particular instance. However, the *best* way to ensure that your partner will quickly receive help is to call for assistance yourself. The only way you can do this is to back away from the danger zone, remain in the unit, and provide the dispatcher with all the needed information. You should discuss this type of situation with your partner before it occurs. Then you can come to an agreement that the uninjured partner will back off a safe distance and call for help. When you have a plan in place, it is easier to face any emergency.

Backing Away from the Scene

Every emergency services response team needs a plan that describes what each team member will do if a situation turns violent.

Certain instances require the driver of the unit to back away from the scene of a vehicle-approach:

- When high-threat weapons are observed
- When the occupants of the vehicle become unruly
- When all of the occupants exit the vehicle and approach the unit and no one appears to need emergency care
- When the incident scene is in a police hot zone
- When your partner has been incapacitated

Until the OIC completes the approach to the vehicle and ensures that the scene is safe, the driver remains behind the wheel of the unit. The driver is responsible for watching the overall scene and the interior of the vehicle for any unusual activity. If something looks suspicious, the driver uses a prearranged signal, such as the backup alarm, to warn the rescuer to return to the unit at once. If circumstances prevent the rescuer from immediately returning to the unit, the driver straightens the wheels of the unit and quickly backs to a safe area.

Be aware that aggressors will probably advance toward the unit as you back away; they usually will not follow on foot for more than 50' because they do not want to leave their vehicle. If they continue to come toward you, you should continue to back away. If necessary, continue backing up until the aggressors return to their vehicle. Remain at a safe distance until help arrives or until the aggressors leave the scene. Backing the unit to safety gives you a constant view of the overall scene, moves the unit out of the danger zone, and makes a call for assistance possible (**Figure 4-8**).

You should avoid driving forward to escape a dangerous situation for several reasons:

- Driving forward momentarily places your unit in the kill zone as you pass the stopped vehicle. The occupants of the vehicle have already attempted aggressive action against you. This gives them a second opportunity to harm you.
- The occupants of the stopped vehicle can follow you.
- Attempting to pull out into the flow of traffic may slow or even stop your forward motion.

Remember that you are the OIC if you are seated in the front passenger seat. When you leave the unit to approach a stopped vehicle, you should close the passenger-side door. If you leave the door open, the side mirror will be out of position and the driver will lose rear visibility on the right side of the unit. The closed door adds to the time it takes you to get back in the unit. However, it enables the driver to back up the unit as soon as you begin your retreat.

If two or more units respond to an incident, placement of later-arriving units is important. If the second unit parks immediately behind the first, it blocks the first unit's escape route. This forces members of the first unit to modify their retreat. They may have to get out of the unit and run past the second unit to use it for protection. This can be avoided if all other arriving units remain a minimum of 50' behind the first unit.

Justifications for Backing Away

Backing away from a dangerous situation is not the same as leaving the scene. Back a safe distance away from the perceived threat, call for law enforcement assistance, and wait at that location until the scene is declared safe for you to begin or continue treatment. You must not

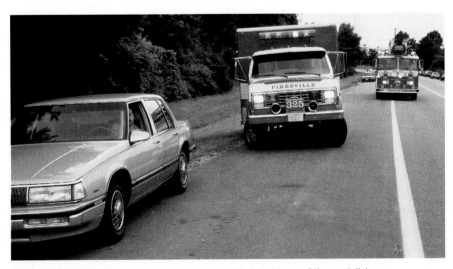

Figure 4-8 Backing away from the scene gives you the advantages of time and distance.

leave the scene until you *know* all occupants of the vehicle require no further medical treatment.

Whenever you back away from a scene, obtain a report from the law enforcement agency that has jurisdiction over the incident scene. Any incident involving aggressive action against the emergency services responders (no matter how minor the threat or how successful the intended aggression) requires a report. Pressing charges against the aggressor is not essential, but the police report provides critical backup documentation on an incident if the patient takes legal action at a later date. The report must clearly explain why you took such an action and include any acts of physical or verbal aggression carried out against you. Note in the report that you felt uncomfortable with the situation, so you backed off in self-defense to wait for law enforcement assistance.

Calling for Assistance

If you need to call for assistance, you must remain calm and professional throughout the entire exchange of information. Make your transmissions clear, concise, and complete. The dispatcher will ask for the "Nature of request for police?" and then repeat everything that you said. If your partner is down, do not worry about using the proper code. In most emergency services communications, plain language is far better than code. Tell the dispatcher, "My partner has just been shot, send the police!" Be ready to provide additional information.

You may have heard about "Signal 13," the universal law enforcement code for "officer down." However, this code cannot be used until your department establishes interagency cooperation with the law enforcement community and all personnel are thoroughly indoctrinated in when to use the code. Signal 13 is used *only* if personnel are in mortal danger.

If you attempt to transmit a Signal 13 before all fire department and emergency medical services field personnel and dispatchers are trained in its use and an interagency agreement exists with the law enforcement community, you may get one or both of the following ineffectual responses:

- The fire department or emergency medical services dispatcher who receives the call will question you about the "nature of the Signal 13," so the police can be told.
- The law enforcement dispatcher will require a detailed explanation of the requested signal before sending the needed assistance.

When you call for help, do not give the dispatcher the location of the vehicle and the aggressor. Instead, provide an exact location where you can meet the law enforcement team. Suggest that they approach your location using a route that avoids the scene of the incident. Make certain that the law enforcement personnel responding to your call are aware that violence has erupted. *Never send an unknowing law enforcement officer into a dangerous situation that you have already left.*

Once the dispatcher acknowledges your call for assistance, you must supply the following information:

- The number of aggressors involved
- The number and type of injuries
- The number and type of weapons involved
- The make, color, body style, and license number of the vehicle involved
- The direction of travel if the vehicle leaves the scene before the law enforcement personnel arrive

Whenever a unit in the field requests law enforcement assistance because of violence, the dispatcher should automatically send an additional emergency medical services unit and a supervisor to the location of the unit requesting assistance. Additional units should not be sent to the original location of the incident, which is now the center of the danger zone.

SURVIVAL TIPS

1 Remember that you are on the scene of an incident to help someone in need of assistance. If you lose control of the situation, you lose the ability to provide an acceptable level of service. Return to the unit, and leave the danger zone.

2 Develop a code word that lets your partner know that you've found a weapon on the patient. Make the code something simple such as calling your partner by the wrong name. Select the name in advance and make sure everyone knows it. All team members within hearing distance will instantly recognize the potential danger when they hear the code word.

3 If a patient is armed, you must immobilize the hands. You may be kicked, bitten, or head-butted, but you cannot be shot. Secure the hands and the patient will be unable to reach the weapon.

4 If you take a firearm from a patient, **do not** attempt to unload the weapon. All weapons have different sensitivities. The weapon may have a shaved-down trigger mechanism, or be in the cocked position with the safety "on." If the safety moves to the off position during the accident, the gun may discharge.

5 If the patient becomes violent in the back of the unit, do not try restraint. Stop the unit and get out. Make sure the driver takes the keys and a portable radio. Call for assistance. Treat this situation as if you were backing away from a danger zone. Now, however, the unit is the danger zone, and you must back away to a safe area on foot.

Chapter 5

Residential Incidents

Emergency response personnel are frequently called to residential areas to assist someone injured in an assault or domestic dispute. The experienced responder will automatically exercise caution on any call involving injuries from violent action. But calls that involve violence are not the only ones that require caution. Any call has the potential of becoming a dangerous situation (**Figure 5-1**). In particular, you should question the cause any time you receive a call reporting "severe bleeding." An "attempted suicide" could turn into a homicide, with you as the victim. Do not assume you will find friendly faces at the scene of a "nature unknown" call. Even an innocent "sick person" can unexpectedly become aggressive. A petite, elderly patient can suddenly become violent and powerful as a result of medication toxicity or overdose.

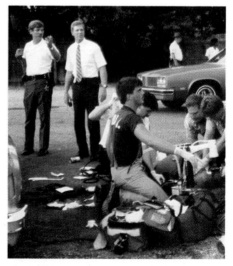

Figure 5-1 When the engine company and paramedic units arrived at this shooting scene before the police, the gunman was still on the parking lot and would not allow them to approach the victim. *(Courtesy Keith R. Hammack, Glen Burnie, MD)*

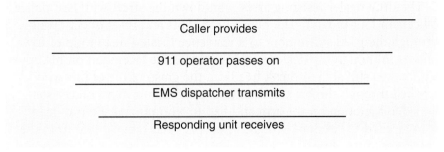

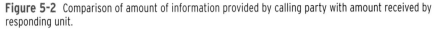

Figure 5-2 Comparison of amount of information provided by calling party with amount received by responding unit.

Many times the caller is too hysterical to provide complete information. Dispatchers should share this detail with you and you should ask yourself, "Why was the caller hysterical?" Until you can answer this question, proceed with caution.

Despite technical advances in communications, you cannot be certain that the information you receive from dispatch is accurate and complete. In many situations the details are repeated several times before they reach the responding unit. Each time a call is filtered, information vital to the responding unit may be omitted or inaccurately recorded. A comparison of the amount of information provided by the caller to that received by the responding unit may resemble an inverted pyramid (**Figure 5-2**).

For example, a caller to 9-1-1 reports "a person having a heart attack in a blue van on the parking lot of Albertson's Market." The 9-1-1 operator relays "heart attack in a van on the parking lot of Albertson's Market" to the EMS dispatcher. The EMS dispatcher sends an Advanced Life Support (ALS) unit to "a heart attack in the parking lot of Albertson's Market." The ALS crew members record and respond to "a heart attack at Albertson's Market." When they arrive, they see more than 50 vehicles of all descriptions in the parking lot and look inside the store for the stricken person.

Never assume that you have adequate information to disregard the potential for danger on any call. Before entering a residence, use a systematic approach to increase your chances of avoiding potentially dangerous situations. The approach technique may not be required on every call, but if you practice and refine it on every response, you will be prepared when a dangerous situation occurs.

An Escalating Incident

The following incident is an example of what can happen to you when you least expect it. As you read the narrative, which was provided by one of the firefighters involved, put yourself in this situation and consider your reactions.

At approximately 6 PM on an early fall evening, the crew from Engine 46 was sitting in the kitchen of its quarters with a visiting police officer. Conversation stopped when the officer's portable radio began to broadcast details of the arrest of a drug dealer. The incident was just about three blocks from the station.

The drug dealer resisting arrest, ran down the street with two police officers in foot pursuit. The police fired shots and the suspect dived through the glass storm door of a residence located in a group of row houses. Although the dealer sustained a massive laceration on his upper leg, he was still able to break free from the grasp of the officer who reached through the broken door and grabbed him. This officer sustained a laceration on the arm and had to stop pursuit. Four officers were needed to subdue the fighting suspect and remove him from the basement of the house.

Medic 14 was dispatched to "assist an injured police officer in a residence, Belvedere Avenue." But by the time the unit arrived, the injured officer had gone to the hospital and the four police officers were struggling to control the dealer, who was bleeding profusely. Before the crew could reach the patient, he collapsed in full cardiac arrest. By this time a substantial crowd had gathered. The people assumed that the man had been beaten into submission by the police, and they started to turn ugly. While assisting the cardiac patient, the medic unit called for an engine company backup.

At this point, Engine 46 received its call to "assist Medic 14 with a cardiac patient in a residence, Belvedere Avenue." The engine company had to work its way through an estimated crowd of 200 angry neighbors to reach the patient. The patient was finally stabilized and transported to the nearest hospital where he later died. Following their procedure for this type of incident, the police stopped all routine patrols within a 6-square-block area surrounding the house on Belvedere Avenue. This action further upset the neighborhood residents.

A fire alarm from a street box was received in the same immediate area at about 8 PM—it was a false alarm. An "unknown type fire" call was received from the same location at about 8:30 PM—it was a trash fire. Both times the engine company encountered large crowds but was able to return to quarters without confrontation.

Shortly after 9 PM, Engine 46 was dispatched to a "Medic standby, unknown type of injured person" at the same residence on Belvedere Avenue. The street appeared quiet, but two patrol cars and four police officers escorted the engine to the location. There, a group of eight adult males awaited the arriving crew. The fire lieutenant, both firefighters, and all four police officers entered the residence to assess the reported patient. When they found no visible injuries, the fire and police personnel returned to the front porch where they met two responders from an arriving medic unit. While they conferred on the previous patient's condition, an unknown assailant began shooting at them. Bullets struck tree limbs 3' over their heads. Everyone dived for cover and scrambled into the house. The police radioed that they were under fire. Even though the shooting continued, the residents of the house ordered all fire and police personnel to leave.

Only the pump operator had remained with the engine. He observed three people enter the house across the street just before the shooting. The operator backed the engine down the street and was turning around when the shots rang out. He notified dispatch that there was trouble at the scene. The battalion chief, unaware that the lieutenant and two firefighters were trapped in the house, ordered the engine to return to quarters immediately.

A police helicopter and a squad of police officers made a sweep down Belvedere Avenue so the crew could exit the house. But because the engine had left the scene, the crew was stranded. They hid behind a group of cars on the parking lot of a nearby supermarket. The sounds of gunshots, breaking glass, and yelling were all around them when the lieutenant radioed for help. After about 20 minutes, a patrol car found and returned the crew to the engine house safely.[1]

Fortunately, these kinds of situations are rare. However, if you were involved in a similar incident, would you be prepared?

Arriving on the Scene

Emergency services units habitually arrive on the scene with flashing lights and wailing sirens. Personnel jump from the unit, fill their arms with equipment, run the length of the sidewalk, and charge through the door with very little thought for their own safety. This approach has no element of surprise; it is more of a "Here we are, where's the patient?" type of arrival.

For your own safety, turn off the siren and warning lights far enough in advance to prevent the occupants of the residence from hearing and seeing your arrival (**Figure 5-3**). If the address is in a subdivision, you can usually turn off the warning lights and sirens when you enter the neighborhood. If the call is on a through street, you can turn them off a couple of blocks before the address. Use the siren only when traffic conditions dictate, when traffic is congested during morning and late afternoon travel. Remember that a siren can be heard from a great distance

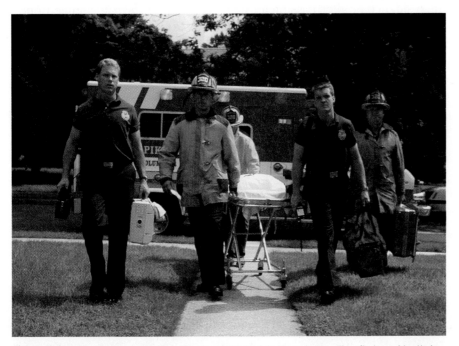

Figure 5-3 Properly prepared paramedics do not charge into the unknown. They first consider their own safety and then that of the patient.

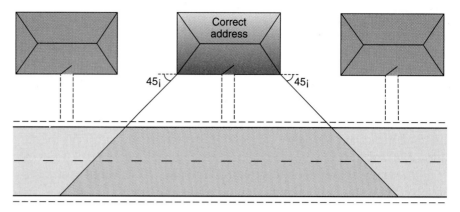

Figure 5-4 To prevent the occupants in the house from observing your arrival, do not stop your unit in the shaded area.

at night. Unnecessary use of the sirens and emergency warning lights will have three results:

- It will eliminate the element of surprise.
- It will damage public relations on legitimate calls. Many people are embarrassed to use emergency services. They appreciate units showing discretion.
- It will draw a crowd when you arrive on the scene. In many areas, having a crowd converge around the unit is not safe.

If you stop the unit directly in front of the structure, the occupants can watch your every move and still remain unseen. Stop the unit approximately 100' from the residence. A rule of thumb is to stop before reaching an imaginary line that runs 45° from the near corner of the residence or after passing an imaginary line of the same angle from the far corner of the residence (**Figure 5-4**). Pulling past the residence is optimal because you can observe three sides of the structure before you leave the unit (**Figure 5-5**). As you approach the residence, you see the near side; as you slowly pass, you see the front; and after you stop the unit, you observe the far side. You need to learn as much as possible

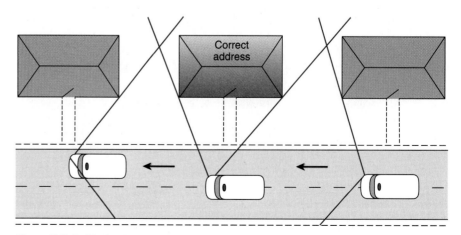

Figure 5-5 Positioning the unit on far side of the residence permits a three-sided observation.

about the situation outside and inside the residence while maintaining your element of surprise (**Figure 5-6**).

Enter long driveways with caution. Position your unit where you probably cannot be seen from the residence (**Figure 5-7**). If no cover is available, position your unit near enough to the residence to provide the required service. If the driveway configuration permits, position the unit in line with the corner of the residence. Finally, turn the unit around to ensure a direct route of exit from the property. Escaping by driving forward is much easier than backing out. If the response is after dark and enough natural light is present, turn the headlights off before entering the driveway. If necessary, use the parking lights to make the approach.

Apartment buildings and townhouse complexes present unique approach problems because of overcrowded parking lots, dead-end streets, and cul-de-sacs. When approaching a multistory apartment building, scan upper-floor windows, patios, and the roof line for signs of a setup. After you complete the scan, do not look straight up; a falling object may strike you in the face. Wear helmet protection whenever you are working near a multistory building.

Many apartment buildings have security doors at the main entrance. People gain entry by ringing the doorbell of the apartment they want to enter, and the occupant unlocks the main entrance door (**Figure 5-8**). To gain access to this type of building and maintain the element of surprise, ring any doorbell *except* the correct one. Use caution on every alarm involving high-density occupancies.

Approaching the Residence

When you properly position the unit, you will be able to approach a residence from an angle. This will keep you out of the normal line of

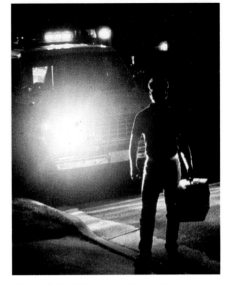

Figure 5-6 Night arrivals dictate that you turn your headlights off before anyone exits the unit to avoid backlighting the rescuer. If you must park the unit on a public street, turn on the parking lights and/or emergency flashers to alert passing motorists.

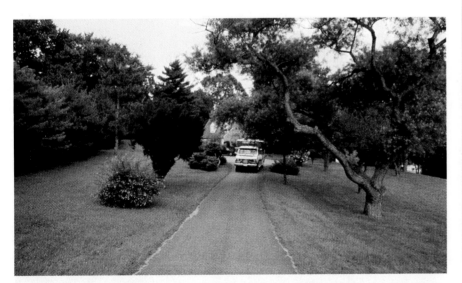

Figure 5-7 A properly positioned medic unit at the end of a long driveway commands a view of two sides of the residence, yet remains out of a direct line with any windows or doors.

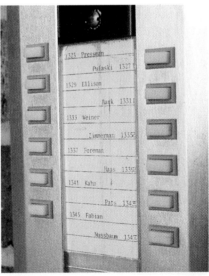

Figure 5-8 Doorbell pushbuttons on the front entrance of an apartment building with a security door.

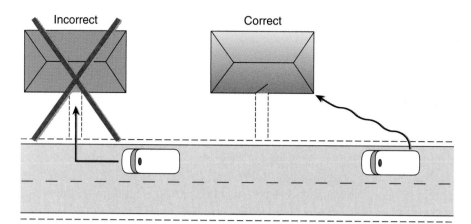

Figure 5-9 Approaching the residence from an angle permits you to maintain the element of surprise.

sight. The occupant will be looking for you to approach from a frontal position and not from across the lawn at an angle (**Figure 5-9**).

Two personnel should be used for residential approaches so that each can watch for the other's safety. In addition, the amount of equipment needed for a residential response is usually more than one person can carry. When removing equipment from the unit, do not slam the compartment doors—shut them quietly.

When you approach the residence, concentrate on the area surrounding the structure (**Figure 5-10**). This is not the time for idle conversation. Use all of your senses to gather information about the incident:

- What do you see when you look through the windows? (Do not stand directly in front of the window. Stand to the side and several steps away from the wall.)
- What do you hear from the inside?
- Do you see or hear a struggle?
- Do you see any high-threat weapons?
- Do you hear loud or abusive voices?
- How many voices are there?
- Do you feel that the environment is safe for you to enter?

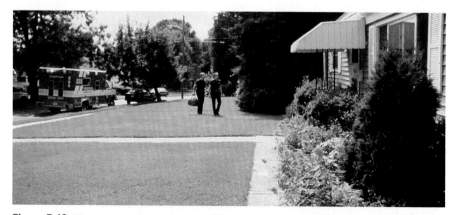

Figure 5-10 When you near the residence, shift your concentration to the structure.

After you reach the front entrance, analyze all the information obtained during the approach before announcing your presence and entering the residence. Do not knock on the door until you are ready to go inside. If you doubt the urgency of the need for medical assistance, perform a scene size-up from the front porch *before* making your presence known. If the occupants are yelling at one another, they are conscious and their airways are patent. If they continue to argue, it is doubtful that either is bleeding profusely, and their need for medical assistance is probably not urgent.

Anytime danger is indicated, abort the approach and back away to the unit. Do not turn your back to the residence—keep the source of your apprehension in sight. Remember, withdrawing to an area of safety is not the same as leaving the scene. Until you have determined that no medical assistance is required, do not leave the scene.

After you are back in the unit, call for law enforcement assistance and move the unit away from the building to an area of relative safety. Inform the dispatcher of the problem and where you will meet the police officers, possibly at the nearest intersection. When they arrive at the scene, brief the officers on the situation before they approach the residence.

SURVIVAL TIPS

1) Before starting the approach, remove all loose items (such as change and keys) from your pockets. You do not want to carry anything unnecessarily noisy that may destroy your element of surprise.

2) While in the unit, keep the unit radio's volume level just loud enough for clear communications. Start each response and approach with the volume on portable radios turned very low. Increase the volume only when needed.

3) Determine if the attempted suicide is a *medical suicide* or a *traumatic suicide* before arriving on the scene. A person who has swallowed a bottle of pills is usually not going to hurt you; however, the person who had an unsuccessful suicide attempt using a weapon may turn that weapon on you.

4) On a reported shooting, stabbing, or traumatic suicide, consider stopping the unit a block or more before the address. Remain with the unit until law enforcement personnel arrive on the scene and declare the area safe.

5) A person who requests assistance from emergency services does not have a "signed contract." If you feel your personal safety is endangered, you are under no obligation to enter the residence.

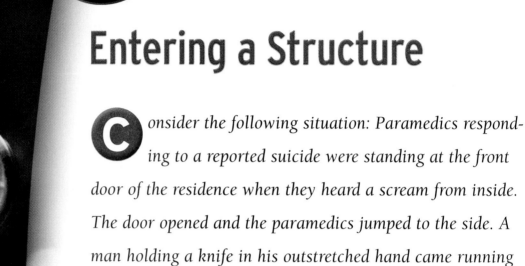
Entering a Structure

Consider the following situation: Paramedics responding to a reported suicide were standing at the front door of the residence when they heard a scream from inside. The door opened and the paramedics jumped to the side. A man holding a knife in his outstretched hand came running out of the house. If the paramedics had not taken such quick action, one of them might have been stabbed.

Doors and doorways present several opportunities for violence against rescuers. A door does not need to be open to expose you to a hazardous situation. People can fire weapons through closed doors in an attempt to injure the person on the other side (**Figure 6-1**). Veteran police officers and paramedics advise new personnel not to position

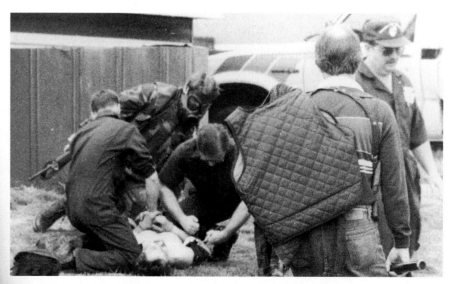

Figure 6-1 Paramedics and SWAT personnel care for a man who had fired an arrow through a closed door at approaching paramedics. *(Courtesy Allen Hafner, Howard County Police Department, Ellicott City, MD)*

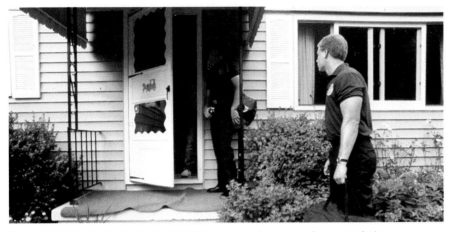

Figure 6-2 Stand on the doorknob side of the entrance when announcing your arrival.

themselves in front of any door, closed or open, until all safety checks are completed and the response team is ready to enter the structure.

Positioning at the Door

The front door to most homes opens inward. When you approach a door, stand to the doorknob side of the entrance to announce your presence (**Figure 6-2**). The occupant should open the door far enough to look around the jamb and see you. If you stand on the hinged side of the door, the occupant can observe you by opening the door only slightly and you would have a limited view of conditions inside the room (**Figure 6-3**). Always stand in a line with the door frame rather than with the plasterboard wall. Door frames are usually constructed of wood or metal and offer better protection than plasterboard

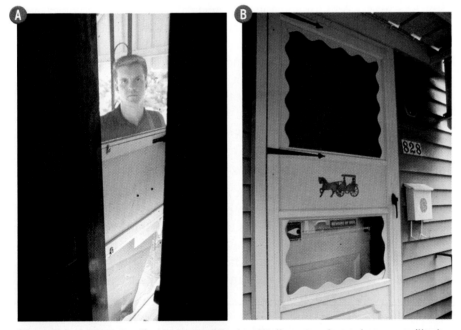

Figure 6-3 If you stand on the hinged side of the door **(A)**, the occupants can observe you without exposing themselves **(B)**.

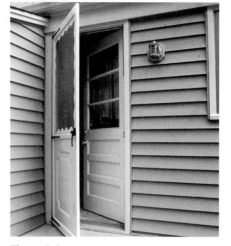

Figure 6-4 Some outer doors are hinged on the opposite side of the door frame as the primary door. Remain on the doorknob side of the primary door when establishing initial contact with the occupants.

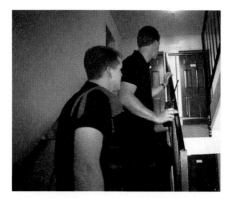

Figure 6-5 When construction features prevent you from standing to the side of the entrance, quickly move down the stairs after knocking on the door.

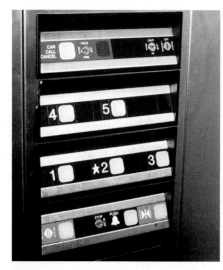

Figure 6-6 Typical elevator control panel.

when a bullet is fired through the wall. If the entryway includes an outer door (a screen or storm door), remain on the doorknob side of the door that opens inward (**Figure 6-4**).

If the call is to a typical three-story apartment building or to a high-rise building, you may not be able to stand to the side of the door because of stairwell or other construction features. One option is to knock on the door and quickly move several steps away before announcing yourself (**Figure 6-5**). Wait until the occupant opens the door and acts appropriately before you return to the front of the door.

When you must use an elevator to reach the apartment, set it on manual or fireman's service (**Figure 6-6**). Silence the alarm before ascending, and hold the car on the floor of the medical emergency (with the door open) until all members of the team are ready to descend. Locate any stairwells before entering the elevator. Visualize their location in relation to the elevator. You may need to use the stairs as an alternate means of escape. When you reach the proper floor, check the stairwell doors and make sure they are unlocked and free to open before you knock on the door of the apartment that reported the emergency.

If the entrance door to the residence is open on your arrival, do *not* go inside without permission; knock and wait to be admitted. It is important to wait because:

- Entering a residence without permission can be considered trespassing or breaking and entering.
- You may be in the wrong location.
- It may be a setup. If you are intentionally lured into a violent environment, you may be seriously injured or killed.

Knock on the door and announce, "Paramedics," "Fire department," or "Rescue squad." Wait for someone to come to the door before you move into the door opening. If someone calls, "come in," without coming to the door, be wary. Ask the person to step outside and talk with you before you enter. If the person says he or she cannot come to the door, find out why. Try to get the occupant to move into your line of sight. If the person refuses without a good reason, consider withdrawing to the unit and requesting law enforcement assistance. If the injured person claims to be alone and unable to come to the door, proceed with caution.

Moving Through the Entrance Way

When your team decides to enter the residence, move without hesitation. Do not pause in the entrance opening. Law enforcement personnel refer to the opening to any room as the *kill zone* (**Figure 6-7**). The occupants can watch the entrance without moving, but you have to turn your head to see the entire room. The time it takes you to locate and recognize a dangerous situation from the entryway may not be enough to save you from a fatal injury.

The first rescuer to enter the residence should look between the door frame and the hinge side of the door while opening the door as far as possible. If the door does not open fully, someone may be hiding behind it. If you are in doubt, do not enter the room.

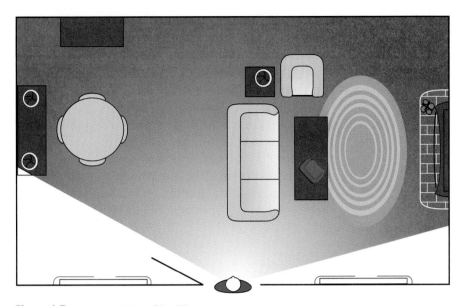

Figure 6-7 An overhead view of the kill zone.

Usually, the last rescuer who enters the residence closes the door out of respect for the occupant. However, you should leave the door ajar if the exact location of the incident was unclear at the time of the call (**Figure 6-8**). Additionally, if you question the continued stability of the incident, leave the door partially open so that other emergency response teams can hear inside the residence before entering.

Moving Within the Structure

Ask the occupant to lead you to the patient. Let the occupant go first through the residence. This will give you the quickest route to the patient and protect you from an unexpected attack. The occupant unknowingly acts as a shield for your team members and gives you a few extra moments to react if the situation deteriorates.

The person who answers the door is usually a family member or close friend of the patient. If this person leads the team to the patient, he or she can help reduce the anxiety level of the patient. The patient is already nervous because of the emergency and will feel reassured if a familiar face comes into the room before several strangers with their arms full of ominous-looking equipment. The following example illustrates the advantage of following the occupant to the patient:

A woman called for an ambulance because her husband was having difficulty breathing. She met the paramedics at the front door with a worried look on her face, pointed to the stairs, and said, "He's in the bedroom." The paramedics ran up the stairs, hurried into the bedroom without knocking, and slid to a stop when the man rolled out of bed, pointing a 9-mm semiautomatic pistol at them. His wife had not told him she was calling the fire department! All he knew was that two strangers had burst unannounced into his bedroom. If the paramedics had asked the wife to take them to the bedroom, this potentially violent encounter could have been prevented.

If the victim has a trauma injury, do not let other occupants in the residence out of your sight until you determine who or what caused the

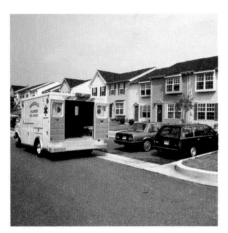

Figure 6-8 Someone will probably be waiting for the first unit on the scene, which will help them identify the correct residence. Following units may not have this assistance.

injury. In one incident, paramedics treating a man with multiple stab wounds to the abdomen asked the patient who stabbed him. The patient pointed over the paramedic's shoulder and said, "She did." The paramedics turned to see the woman who had met them at the front door standing between them and the door with a large knife in her hand.

If one of the occupants in the room with the patient starts to leave (no matter what the reason), a member of the rescue team should accompany the person. If you cannot follow the person, say that you need assistance with the patient and ask the person to perform a small task that will keep the person in the room and within your line of sight. This reduces the possibility of the person obtaining a weapon and returning to the scene.

Weapons in the Residence

As you proceed to the patient's location, scan the rooms you are passing through for weapons. Make a mental note of the location of both high-threat and low-threat weapons (see Chapter 3). When you reach the patient, pay particular attention to weapons that may be within the patient's reach (**Figure 6-9**). Move scissors, knitting needles, ashtrays, fireplace pokers, and other dangerous articles out of the patient's reach to make room for your equipment. Whenever possible, place sharp objects under furniture or between cushions. Avoid touching or moving high-threat weapons such as guns and knives; the weapon may have been used in a crime and, if you pick it up, you may destroy irreplaceable evidence. If you see a gun or a knife, move the patient away from the weapon rather than moving the weapon away from the patient. Use an excuse, such as lack of light or room, for your action.

More potential weapons are found in a kitchen than in any other room in a residence. These weapons are within easy reach from any part of most kitchens. If you must provide patient care in a kitchen, be extremely alert to the possibilities for injury.

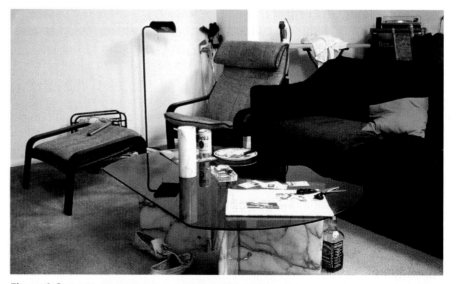

Figure 6-9 Identify the possible threats to your safety in this scene.

Today, many people keep loaded firearms in the house for personal protection. A nightstand next to the bed, a dresser drawer, or an end table next to a favorite chair in the family room are popular locations to conceal these weapons. You may not see a weapon but, for your own safety, assume it is there. Many people who own weapons have no training in the proper use of firearms. The weapon may be poorly constructed or need repair. A round may be in the chamber, and the safety mechanism, if it has one, is probably off. For your own safety, avoid picking up a gun.

Do not pick up a weapon and put it in the jump kit or drug box for safekeeping. The weapon is not your property, and you do not have the authority to remove it from a residence. If you put the weapon in your equipment, you can be charged with stealing, no matter how innocent the action or how sincere your intentions. If you must move a weapon, make a mental note of its original location. Give this information to the police officer writing the report and mention the location on your incident report. Always inform law enforcement personnel of the location of all firearms you have found in the residence.

If you are aware of the potential presence of firearms within a residence, you will be prepared to make timely and effective decisions regarding patient treatment.

SURVIVAL TIPS

1. If the person who opens the door is belligerent, you are not obligated to enter. Do not try to gain entry when you are met with hostility.

2. Always move *down* the stairs (away from the door) when waiting for someone to open a door. If you move up the stairs and violence erupts, you will not have an avenue of escape.

3. Attempt a window entry to a residence only after all other conventional methods have failed. The occupant may see you as a threat and take aggressive action against you. If you must enter through a window, always stand to the side of the opening and shout, "Fire department," "Rescue squad," or "Paramedics," several times before entering.[1]

4. Do not allow a person who has been involved in a dispute with the victim to assist with patient care; this may precipitate further violence. Use caution when asking other residents or occupants for assistance in packaging the patient.

5. Whenever possible, avoid treating a patient who is within reach of any weapon. Either move the weapon (if it is a low-threat) or move the patient (preferred action).

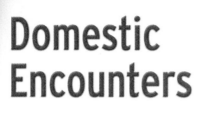

Domestic Encounters

Domestic disturbances are among the most dangerous situations faced by law enforcement officers. Emergency services personnel must be aware of the dangers involved and handle these incidents with extreme caution. Consider this example:

On a late spring evening, a man in New Lancaster Valley, Pennsylvania, reported that he had been assaulted by his son during a domestic dispute and requested the police. A short time later, a structure fire was reported at the same location. As the responding police and fire personnel approached the house, they were fired upon from inside. Before they could reach safety, one firefighter was killed and another firefighter and a state trooper were wounded.[1] The wounded firefighter died four days later.[2] Although the situation seemed calm when emergency services personnel arrived, it escalated into a deadly situation in a matter of seconds. The same thing could happen during your next response to a domestic dispute.

If a violent or physical dispute is in progress when you arrive at a residence, wait for law enforcement assistance before you enter. Sometimes tempers subside when the rescue team arrives on the scene and flare up again after you start patient care. When this happens, separate the fighting parties as quickly as possible, but do not stand between them (**Figure 7-1**). Use voice commands, eye contact, and body language to manipulate

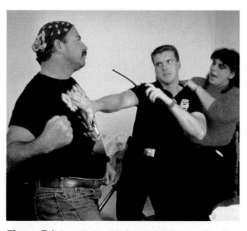

Figure 7-1 Do not stand between fighting parties. You may be the one who receives the most injuries.

the people to turn away from each other until they can no longer see each other. The tension level will go down if the individuals involved in the dispute are no longer facing each other.

Calm the Situation with Voice Control

Your voice is the most effective tool you can use to keep out of trouble in a dispute. Knowing what words to use or not use in a situation is only part of your goal. You must also be aware of the tone, pacing, pitch, and rhythm of your voice.

Be careful in choosing your words; certain words may further antagonize the person you are trying to calm. Do not use condescending or overtly familiar terms such as "sport," "buddy," or "pal." Certainly terms such as "gramps," "little lady," "grandma," and "pop" are inappropriate when speaking with older people. You may use other phrases without even thinking about the effect they may have. The phrase "calm down," for instance, is often heard at emergency scenes, whether the emergency is a serious illness or a domestic argument. Generally, such words do nothing to calm someone whose emotions are high and may do more to inflame the situation. A better phrase to use would be, "we will do our best to help."

Individuals involved in domestic situations may not be thinking clearly due to their elevated anxiety levels. Using the wrong word may cause aggression to be directed toward you. Remain calm and impartial. By empathizing with the individuals, you will further defuse the situation. This does not mean you necessarily sympathize with either party; you are merely looking at the problem through their eyes.

Only a small portion of a message is carried by the words you use. Much more meaning is conveyed by four elements within the voice: tone, pace, pitch, and modulation.[3] The tone of your voice is obviously important and must match the situation. A tone of command or authority is certainly appropriate if you are the Incident Commander at an

---

Box 7-1: **Phrases to Avoid**

Come here!

What do you want me to do about it?

Those are the rules.

You got a problem?

It's none of your business!

Calm down!

This is for your own good.[4]

emergency. But that same hard-nosed tone of voice and facial expression would do little to defuse a domestic argument. Even though you may be having a rotten day, you cannot let your voice show your frustration. The pace of your voice relates to its speed. You alter the pitch of your voice by adjusting it higher or lower. Even the rhythm and inflection, or modulation, can alter the meaning you give to the words you use.

Talk to people with the same respect that you expect from them, regardless of your personal opinion of them. Avoid talking up to people, as if they were on a higher social level, as well as talking down to people, as if they were children. If you treat someone with little or no respect, that person may turn on you and the situation can quickly deteriorate to a dangerous level. For example, when you introduce yourself, ask the person, "What's your name?" If the answer gives you both first and last name such as "Mike Smith," respond by asking, "Do you mind if I call you Mike?" It is more appropriate to address older people by their surnames such as Mr. Smith or Mrs. Jones.

Conduct yourself as a professional in a business environment. Your duty is to act in a professional manner, no matter how unpleasant or difficult the situation may be. Start when you knock on the front door. Introduce yourself, "Hi, I'm Bob Jones from Anytown EMS. How can I help?" Wipe your feet before you enter a residence to show respect for the person's home. Once inside, if you find yourself involved in a domestic argument, separate and keep the occupants individually engaged in conversation while your partner evaluates the patient. A good way to engage the occupants is to enlist their help in obtaining a history about the patient. Because your objective is to identify the person who needs emergency medical care and transport that person to a medical facility, you can ask questions such as, "What is her height and weight? Does she have a medical history? Any allergies? Any family medical conditions?" Be creative and give your partner enough time to do the initial assessment and initiate care. Your attention to detail and your professionalism can make the difference between a successful and an unsuccessful situation.

At an emergency scene, you may be confronted by family members who are preventing you from delivering quick, efficient patient care. Simply put, they are getting in the way. Your urge to yell, "Move!" or "Get out of the way!" punctuated by a few curse words may be understandable. It may even result in the desired effect. However, it will leave a bad feeling behind you. The smart emergency medical technician or firefighter will explain the need or benefits of complying with a request by saying something like, "If you move back, we can help your brother and get him to a hospital quickly." A stronger phrase may be used when the above phrase is ineffective. You may say, for example, "If you don't let us help your brother, he may die." By letting the person know what could happen, you allow him or her to further consider the actions. Remember, voluntary compliance can be gained more often when you explain, "why." Taking a few seconds to explain the situation to a family member or bystander can be more effective and leave a better impression of your service than simply shouting orders.

Turn the Individual with Eye Contact

Speak and establish eye contact with one of the individuals involved in the dispute. After you make eye contact, continue talking to this individual and slowly move in a circular direction away from the other person (**Figure 7-2**). If the individual is also focused on you, he or she will turn with you and away from the other person. Your partner should be doing the same thing with the other person but moving in the opposite direction. Eventually, the two parties will have their backs to one another and calming them should be easier. Showing concern and empathy aids in gaining the person's attention and confidence. Do not grab and turn the person; a discreet movement of your eyes and body will give the desired effect.

When you execute this movement, be sure that you do not unintentionally place yourself in a tactically unsound position. One common mistake is to move the person into a position between you and your primary or secondary escape route (**Figure 7-3**).

Do not lose sight of your partner during this move. Use your peripheral vision to watch all other activity in the area (**Figure 7-4**), as you continue the conversation with the individual. If you see a weapon in the waistband or back pocket of the other person's trousers, warn your partner by using a prearranged code word, such as calling your partner by the wrong name.

Body Language

The way you stand when talking to the disputing parties will influence the situation. If you enter a room and assume an aggressive posture (such as with feet apart and hands on your hips), you invite abuse. Standing with your arms crossed over your chest may also bring a challenge from one of the involved parties. This gesture conveys the mes-

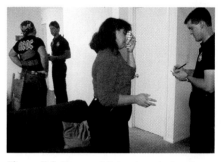

Figure 7-2 If you maintain eye contact and conversation with the individual as you begin to move, the participant will likely move wherever you lead.

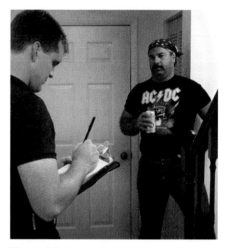

Figure 7-3 Do not allow any of the participants in the dispute to position themselves between you and the door.

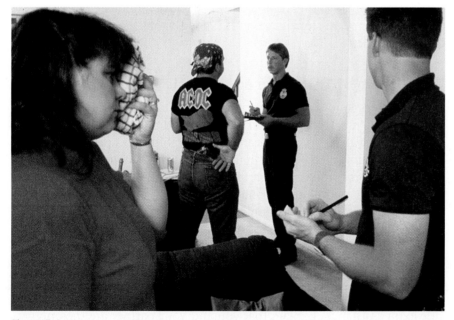

Figure 7-4 Using your peripheral vision, look for weapons on the individual your partner is interviewing.

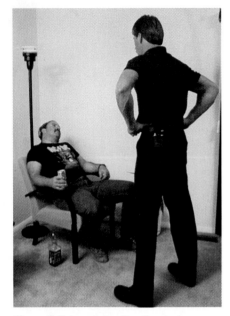

Figure 7-5 Do not stand in a threatening or indifferent position.

sage, "My mind is made up; I cannot be swayed" (**Figure 7-5**). Using an interview stance in these situations is nonthreatening and provides you with a high degree of safety.

The amount of space between you and the other party is also significant. Honoring an individual's personal space is a sign of respect. But remember that various cultures have different dimensions for personal space. As you may be aware, most European cultures are comfortable with about 6' of personal space between people. However, personal space requirements in Middle Eastern cultures are slightly less. People of Asian descent are more comfortable with a space of more than 6' between individuals. Defending against aggressive movements toward you is discussed in Chapter 13.

Buttons

Everyone has at least one "button"—a sensitive area that triggers an angry response. Know what annoys *you*. Take a moment to write down those things that may cause you to lash out. Maybe it's the person who spits on you or the one who says, "I pay your salary." Perhaps you tend to shove the inconsiderate person who does not move out of your way as you attempt to reach a patient. If you can identify your buttons, you will be able to recognize them and be less likely to let them influence your behavior on the scene.

Verbal insults by patients, family members, or bystanders are common. The words used carry only the weight that you give to them. Responding to one insult with another will only invite a counterattack and may also result in a physical confrontation.

If someone pushes your button, back off and try to remain calm. Control your encounters and do not react to these situations. If you lose control, you may be drawn into a confrontation with the patient or others associated with the incident. Do not allow yourself to fall into this trap. If you remain calm and in control of your emotions, you will maintain your professionalism and feel good about the way you handled the incident.

Tier System of Entry into an Unstable Area

All units responding to an emergency rarely arrive at the same time. In most incidents, unequal travel distances and delays associated with interagency notification may mean that several minutes pass between the arrival of units. This generally results in a tier system of entry.

Even if several units arrive on the scene at the same time, the tier entry system should be used (**Figure 7-6**). This gives the occupants an opportunity to adjust to your presence. If everyone walks through the door at the same time, the residents may feel overwhelmed. This could result in a potentially violent situation if the incident involves a domestic dispute.

If you are part of the first crew to arrive, tell the occupants that additional personnel will be coming to bring additional equipment or provide extra assistance. Explain that you and your partner are the only crew members who will be dealing with the occupants; all other per-

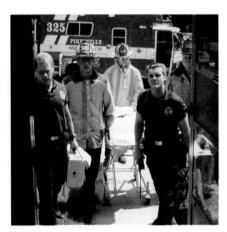

Figure 7-6 Using a tier system of entry prevents the occupants from feeling they are being invaded.

sonnel will remain outside or out of the way unless they are needed to assist in treatment.

If you are on a later arriving unit, knock on the door and wait for permission to enter. If the first unit has managed to settle the domestic argument and separate the parties, your unexpected entry may start the argument all over again. This time the anger may be aimed at you, and you will have to start at the beginning to calm the people, explain your presence, and separate the fighting parties.

Using Barriers to Separate Individuals

Physical obstacles such as coffee tables and sofas may also serve as psychological barriers to an ongoing fight. Although it is easy to jump over or walk around most furniture, these objects can be used to successfully separate the antagonists (**Figure 7-7**). Other construction features such as curtain walls, room dividers, and breakfast bars can also separate people. Large items may block the line of sight between the fighting parties, which automatically calms the situation. It is difficult to continue fighting with someone who cannot be seen. However, if you use these barriers to separate the fighting parties, be sure to position yourself where you can see your partner (**Figure 7-8**). You want to be able to cover each other in the event something happens.

Distraction Techniques

Sometimes a domestic dispute will flare up after you have successfully separated the parties. Often one person thinks the other person is telling you something that is not true or is requesting you to pass a message to the police. If the individual that you are treating or interviewing suddenly turns away from you and starts yelling at the other person, quickly employ a distraction technique to break the person's train of thought. Do this as soon as possible to prevent the argument from escalating to its original level.

For example, you could tell the person that your pen ran out of ink and ask for another one so you can write down some necessary information. You could ask to see a driver's license or an insurance card for billing. If you start talking about sending a bill for your services, you will usually get the person's undivided attention. Ask unnecessary questions that require more than a "yes" or "no" answer. Always write down the answers; this will buy you time while your partner works with the other person involved in the dispute.

Distraction techniques are also useful if the person you are treating attempts to leave the room. Request that the person stay because you are almost finished with the interview. The claim, "I only want to get a pack of cigarettes," can be countered with, "We prefer that you not smoke right now because we have oxygen in the room." If the person insists, follow and continue to ask questions about the incident. Depending on the severity of the disagreement, the person may be going after a weapon to continue the dispute (**Figure 7-9**). Your presence may discourage this possibility. If you see the person get a weapon, run back to warn your partner and the patient that the situation may explode. *Leave the residence immediately!*

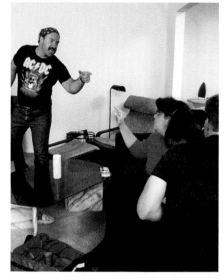

Figure 7-7 Furniture is a barrier between the parties.

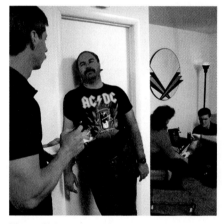

Figure 7-8 Never lose sight of your partner when separating fighting parties.

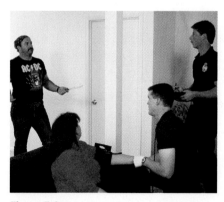

Figure 7-9 Do not permit anyone to leave the room alone; the person may return with a weapon.

Avoiding the Violent Situation

If the person adamantly refuses to allow you to follow, do not insist to the point that causes violence to erupt. Permit the person to leave while you stay with your partner and the patient. As soon as the person is out of sight, you and your partner should leave the residence. If possible, take the patient with you. If the patient hesitates or starts to argue, leave the patient behind. Do not gather your equipment; exit the residence and call for law enforcement assistance from a safe location.

Tell the dispatcher where to have police meet your unit (possibly at the nearest intersection) so that you can explain the situation. Do not allow police officers to proceed to the residence without first attempting to inform them of the conditions inside (**Figure 7-10**). They were probably told to, "assist EMS on a domestic," and may not know that you have already been in the residence. Explain to the officers what happened when you knocked on the door, what was said inside, what you saw, how many people were present, and what caused you to leave the house and call for assistance. If you were unable to bring the patient out with you, advise the officers that a patient requiring emergency medical treatment is still in the house. Request that they secure the residence so that you can safely return to your patient and continue care.

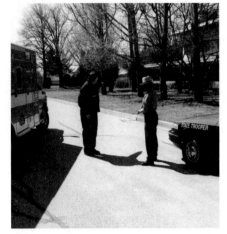

Figure 7-10 Do not send the local police to the house without first informing them of the nature of the call.

The officers will probably call for backup before proceeding. When this happens, remain where you are and wait for the additional units to arrive. Do not approach or reenter the building until law enforcement personnel have secured the scene and declared the residence safe.

There are valid reasons for backing away from a motor vehicle incident, as discussed in Chapter 4. The same criteria apply to backing away from a hostile situation in a building. It should be difficult to convict you of abandoning your patient if you document on your report that you did the following:

- Feared for your personal safety because civilian personnel on the scene were uncooperative and refused to follow your instructions.
- Acted in self-defense.
- Did not take the time to gather up your equipment before leaving the hostile area.
- Left the hostile area at the same time as all other emergency service personnel.
- Did not leave the scene, only the hostile area.
- Called for law enforcement assistance. (Attach a copy of the police report to your report; if not available, include the police case number in your report.)
- Returned to the patient and continued treatment as soon as the area was declared safe by on-scene law enforcement personnel.

In a potentially violent situation, it is important that you and your partner always act as a team. You should agree in advance that if either of you feels that it is time to leave a potentially hostile area, you both will leave at the same time. At some time in your career, you may have to appear in court to testify why you believed that remaining in the area placed you in imminent danger. You will need to explain the explosive nature of the situation and emphasize how you feared for your personal safety. If the defense attorney asks, "What did your partner do?" and you have to reply, "My partner stayed in the house," your judgment may be challenged. Consider how you would respond to the defense attorney's next question: "Why was it too dangerous for you to continue to treat my client, but your partner was able to stay and continue to treat the ex-spouse?" Remember, if it's bad enough for one to leave, it's bad enough for all to leave.

SURVIVAL TIPS

1. Settling domestic disputes is not your responsibility. Your job is to provide prehospital emergency care. If care is not needed, return to service.

2. Most emergency service workers are not trained as marriage counselors, psychologists, psychiatrists, priests, or preachers. Crisis intervention is not part of your job description and should be left to the professionals.

3. Most of your success in speaking to people has to do with the way the message is delivered.

4. Respond to situations; do not react to them.

5. Never let anyone stand between you and your primary escape route.

6. Do not back yourself into a corner.

7. Plan your route of escape before you need it.

8. If violence has occurred in the residence, law enforcement personnel should enter first. Fire and medical personnel enter only after the area is declared safe.

9. Shootings, stabbings, and traumatic suicides are primarily police matters.

10. If the situation deteriorates, leave the building. Meet law enforcement personnel at a secure location and advise them of the situation.

11. A dead emergency medical technician is a useless emergency medical technician.

Chapter 8

Barroom Situations

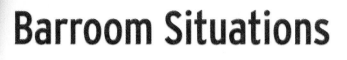

Every city has a district that is noted for problems. When the dispatcher announces an address in this district, everyone hearing the call reacts. Most are thankful that they do not have to respond, but others feel chills up their spines and knots in their stomachs as they hurry to their units.

The address may not be a barroom or the local "knife-and-gun club." Difficult situations are also encountered in sophisticated nightclubs, casinos, crowded restaurants, and even churches. Any location where crowds gather can create difficulties for fire and rescue personnel.

The problems vary from the potential for extreme personal danger to the ridiculous situation that hinders patient care. Consider the case of a waiter in an expensive restaurant who had a heart attack at the height of the dinner hour. When the medic crew arrived, they found the waiter in full cardiac arrest on the floor next to a table. As the paramedics provided emergency life support, other waiters continued to step over the patient's legs and the defibrillation unit, and diners at neighboring tables continued to eat as if nothing had happened.

Consider the danger if this situation occurred in the local knife-and-gun club establishment. A simple request to the bartender to turn down the music so that you could take a blood pressure reading could trigger a violent response from other customers. What would you do then?

Size-Up

Your preparations should begin as soon as you receive the call. Your subconscious reaction to the address starts the information-gathering process. After the dispatcher provides initial to the information, you should follow up with a series of questions. Ask the dispatcher and your partner (particularly if your partner is more familiar with the area than you are):

1. Does this establishment have a history of trouble?
   - Have you personally experienced trouble during calls at this address?
   - Did the trouble endanger your life?
   - Did the trouble interfere with patient care?
2. What is the reported nature of the incident?
   - Did the problem result from natural causes, such as a heart attack?
   - Was the injury accidental or the result of a violent act?
3. If the injury was the result of violence, you need more information before you decide whether to respond immediately, or to wait for law enforcement assistance.
   - Is the person who caused the injury still at the scene?
   - Is violence still occurring?
4. Are the police responding to this call?
   - Are they at the scene?
   - If they are not there yet, what is their estimated time of arrival?

Depending on the location of the call, time of day, and nature of the call, you may need to consider many other questions as well. By gathering information about the call during your trip, you should have enough facts to make a go or no-go decision when you arrive at the scene. If you are not comfortable with the situation when you arrive, wait for police assistance before entering the establishment.

Entering the Establishment

When you decide to enter the building, you can use several tactics to increase your personal safety. If you must enter a dimly lit establishment such as a barroom during daylight hours, you may be unable to see anything inside as your eyes adjust to the loss of light. To partially compensate for the subdued lighting, close one eye, preferably your strong eye, before getting out of your unit. Keep this eye closed as you approach and enter the building. After you are inside, you can open the eye. This eye will already be adjusted to less light, enabling you to see deeper into the dimness.

Do not look directly at objects or people until both eyes have fully adjusted to the light.[1] At first, you will see more clearly with peripheral vision than with direct observation. To use this technique, do not look directly at the object of concern, but look several degrees off-center. Do not fix your gaze on a single object or person; keep your eyes moving around the main object of interest. This increases your off-center vision while your eyes adjust to the available light.

As soon as the door closes behind you and your partner, step to one side of the entrance, if possible (**Figure 8-1**). To prevent anyone from getting behind you, remain close to the wall. Stay in this position and

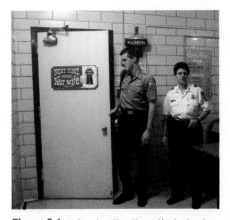

Figure 8-1 Before locating the patient, step to the side of the entrance and size up the room.

assess what you see and hear. Listen to your gut feeling about the emotional temperature of the room as you decide whether to proceed into the building or withdraw to the parking lot and wait for police support. Remember that every situation is different and only the people on the scene can make the decision to proceed or withdraw.

Identify the person who called for assistance. This may be the bartender, the bouncer, or a patron with a cell phone. In many establishments, the bartenders and doormen (bouncers) are the most sober people on the premises. Ask them about the situation. If the patient has been injured in a fight, find out who caused the injury. Is that person still in the building? Was a weapon involved? Where is the weapon?

Contact and Cover

After you locate the patient, use the tactic of "contact and cover." This technique will enable you to keep track of what is occurring around you. One medic assumes the role of care provider and makes "contact" with the sick or injured person. He or she makes a quick assessment using standard emergency care procedures. The second responder begins to gather information about the incident and provides "cover" for the care provider and patient. This responder remains standing while writing down responses to questions or patient information relayed from the contact medic. He or she also monitors the room, continually scanning the area for any signs that tensions are rising (**Figure 8-2**). If the cover person determines that the situation is deteriorating, a subtle nudge to the contact medic should signal that a retreat might be in order.

If the atmosphere starts to become dangerous, you should be prepared to move the patient quickly to safety. An early warning gives you time to be clear of the room before tensions explode. You, your partner, and the patient should remain together as you leave; if you become separated, you may be in greater danger. This technique can be used in a variety of settings, anyplace where violence may erupt.

Never touch anyone in the room except the patient. Depending on a patron's state of sobriety, your actions—no matter how innocent—may be interpreted as an act of aggression or as a move that will belittle the person in the eyes of friends.

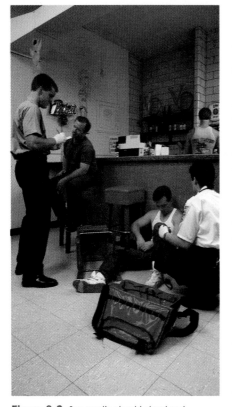

Figure 8-2 One medic should stand and observe the emotional temperature of the room while the other medic assesses the patient.

The Hasty Retreat

In some areas, local protocols emphasize stabilizing and treating patients wherever they are found. Emergency service providers who do not strictly follow this protocol may receive disciplinary action, ranging from a verbal reprimand to a loss of certification, depending on the seriousness of the violation. However, the national trend in patient care is toward rapid evaluation, timely transportation, and stabilization en route to the medical care facility.

When you respond to an incident in a public place, the surroundings may make it difficult for you to provide patient care in the original location. If it will not jeopardize the patient's condition, consider moving the patient out of the public eye. This action will preserve the patient's dignity and avoid additional embarrassment. Anticipate the need to evacuate the patient quickly to an area of safety. If possible, move toward the unit. If not, move to a quieter, less crowded area within the building, or, as last resort, behind the bar or against a wall to wait for assistance.

Before the days of emergency medical technicians, standard procedure was for ambulance personnel to put the patient on a stretcher, place the stretcher in the ambulance, and race for a hospital. Even today, some situations still justify the old swoop-and-scoop tactics. Anyone found in a burning building is usually removed to safety before treatment begins. This action is never questioned as a possible violation of protocol. The imminent danger to the patient and the rescuer justifies immediate removal to a safe location (**Figure 8.3**).

Equally hazardous conditions are found in any public gathering place, especially after a violent act. Treat situations involving violent actions in the same way you treat any other hazardous incident—get in, get the patient, and get out.

In situations where violence suddenly erupts around you, create a diversion by yelling, "Hey, don't throw that!" When your aggressor ducks or turns, run for the door. If possible, take the patient with you.

If the potential for violence is apparent when you enter an establishment, do not stay there. Make a safe retreat by announcing to the room in general, "We need to get the stretcher." Return to the unit and call for police assistance. While waiting for the police to arrive, discuss the situation with your partner, and assemble the equipment you will need to treat the patient. Be ready to enter and start treatment as soon as the police arrive and declare the area safe.

Using Available Human Resources

If the crowd becomes unruly and you believe you will have trouble getting the patient to the door, you have one final option. You can ask for help from the biggest and meanest-looking person in the room—provided that person is not the one who injured your patient. Phrase your request, "We need your help in getting the patient through this crowd. Can you move everybody out of our way?" In this way, you transfer the unmanageable problem of onlooker interference and crowd control to this person. Someone will usually accept the challenge of clearing a path for you.

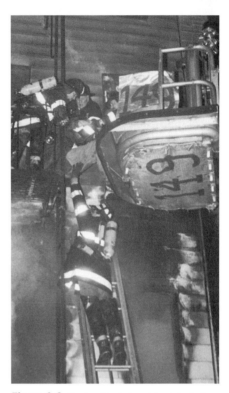

Figure 8-3 Treat patients found in violent situations in the same way you would treat those found in burning buildings–remove the patient to a safe location before starting care. (*Courtesy T. W. McNulty, Fire Department of the City of New York, Randall's Island, NY*)

SURVIVAL TIPS

1 Remember, the information you receive from the dispatcher may not be complete. The "man choking" in the local restaurant may not be a situation involving a foreign object obstructing the airway but an attempted homicide.

2 Never enter a public gathering place without a portable radio. You may need to call for assistance.

3 Never enter a public gathering place alone for a reported trauma injury. There should be a minimum of two rescuers to investigate this type of incident.

4 Never enter an establishment known as a trouble spot without confirming that the police are also responding. Do not assume that the dispatcher notified the police at the time of alarm; always ask!

5 Never enter an establishment if you believe your safety is in question. Notify the dispatcher that you are remaining outside until the police arrive. Allow them to enter and secure the building first.

6 Always document any conditions that force you to move the patient without proper packaging. Emphasize the reasons in your report; for example, "The building was on fire," or "The people were throwing bottles at us."

Chapter 9

Cover and Concealment

In the late afternoon of a hot summer day, the San Diego Fire Department received a report of a shooting incident at a McDonald's restaurant in nearby San Ysidro. The first responding engine was forced to stop short of the scene and the crew had to seek cover behind the engine because of gunfire. The responding battalion chief stopped about 30 yards behind the engine and used his vehicle for cover until the scene was secured by the police department (**Figure 9-1**).[1]

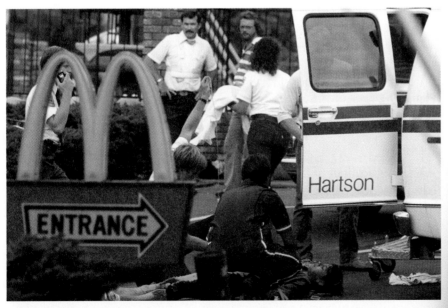

Figure 9-1 Medical personnel treat victim of a massacre at McDonald's restaurant in San Ysidro, California. *(Courtesy Union-Tribune Publishing Co, San Diego, CA)*

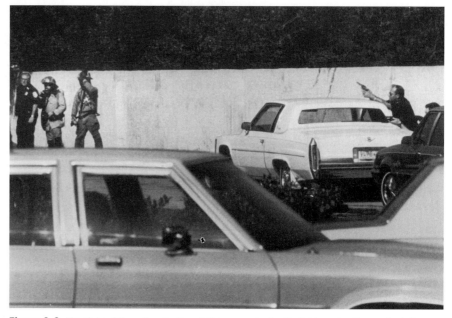

Figure 9-2 The state-of-the-art protective clothing worn by the firefighters standing on the left protects them from heat, not bullets. The police officer would be safer behind the engine block or wheel area. *(Courtesy The Tampa Tribune, Tampa, FL)*

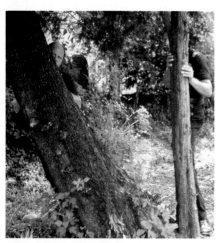

Figure 9-3 Pick a tree that is large enough to conceal all of your body.

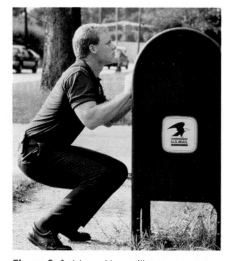

Figure 9-4 A large, blue mailbox on a corner provides cover; the one on a post in front of your house does not.

This example shows the importance of knowing how to use cover and concealment during a violent incident. None of the firefighters was hurt because they had appropriate cover. As you approach an incident, train yourself to scan the area quickly for objects that can provide cover or concealment if violence unexpectedly erupts. Eventually, this will become an automatic procedure, so that you will know where to go for protection. This awareness of your immediate surroundings is vital if an attack occurs, so that you can instinctively locate a safe area. If you fail to react instantly to a sudden attack, you may be seriously injured or killed.

Never assume that you will not be harmed because you are clearly identified as a member of the fire department or an EMS responder. Always assume that the person with the gun will shoot anyone in sight. If the police seek cover, you must not remain in the immediate vicinity (**Figure 9-2**).

Cover

There is a difference between objects that provide cover and those that offer concealment only. Cover objects are usually impenetrable to bullets such as trees, utility poles, mail-collection boxes, dumpsters, curbs, vehicles, and depressions in the ground. When you are using cover, you should make your body conform to the shape of the object as much as possible (**Figure 9-3**). For example, if you crouch behind a mail collection box, you are protected from the knees up, but your ankles and feet remain visible targets. Any part of your body that is exposed can be hit. To minimize exposure, place your feet behind the posts that support the mailbox (**Figure 9-4**).

Assailants who are on higher ground than you (such as in an upper floor window or on a roof) can usually see the upper part of your torso or head over the top of your cover, especially if you are using a wall or motor vehicle as cover (**Figure 9-5**). If this occurs, use the engine block and wheel area of a motor vehicle as cover (see Chapter 2). Avoid the area near the fuel tank, and do not use the area between the wheels as cover. Even though the aggressor cannot see you if you are between the wheels, a skilled shooter can hit you by ricocheting bullets off the pavement in front of you.

Bullets bounce off solid objects at a different angle than the initial hit. When a bullet hits a hard surface (such as a concrete wall or pavement), it flattens out and travels parallel to the surface at a much lower angle (Burke TW, Officer survival: the ricocheting bullet, unpublished data, 1984) (**Figure 9-6**). During the Texas Tower incident in 1966, an ambulance driver was lying behind the ambulance in the area between the wheels. The assailant purposely fired at the ground on the opposite side of the medic unit. The bullets traveled under the unit, struck, and killed the driver.

Select a fire hydrant as cover only if you cannot immediately find a larger objects. You will soon become uncomfortable trying to conform your body to such a small object. You may be shot in the arm, knee, or shoulder, but your central body mass vital organs will be protected. If this is the only cover available, it is better than remaining in the open (**Figure 9-7**).

Items inside a structure and the structure itself can provide either cover or concealment, depending on their construction. Items that can be used for cover, such as a solid oak desk or a refrigerator, can stop a bullet. If you dive behind the sofa or a stuffed chair, you have concealed yourself but are not protected by cover.

Using Walls as Cover

You cannot assume that a wall will provide safe cover. Many walls will provide only concealment. For your safety and survival, you must recognize if the type of wall you have chosen gives you cover or con-

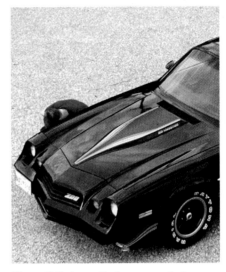

Figure 9-5 An assailant can see part of your body from above your position of cover.

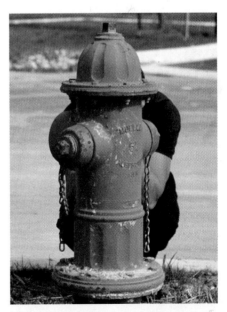

Figure 9-7 Fire hydrants provide excellent cover from bullets, but hiding behind one becomes uncomfortable quickly.

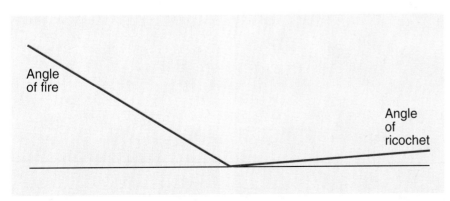

Angle of fire

Angle of ricochet

Figure 9-6 The bullet's angle as it ricochets is much less than that of the original shot.

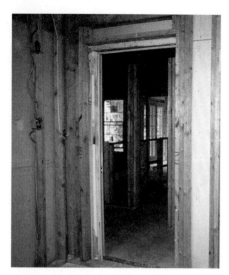

Figure 9-8 The density of wall framing is greater near doors and windows.

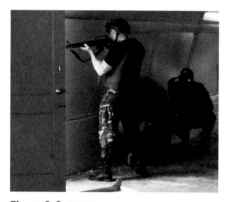

Figure 9-9 SWAT team member uses door frame as cover, while medics use crouch low to gain cover from block wall.

cealment only (**Figure 9-8**). For example, brick or concrete-block walls are much safer than cinder-block walls. The porous nature of cinder-blocks will not absorb the bullet's energy and stop it. However, most interior walls are constructed with wood or aluminum studs and covered with drywall or siding. They may conceal you but are not good cover because they are not impenetrable. If your only protection is behind a frame wall, try to stand near the door or window frames. These areas are usually constructed with extra framing materials and contain more wood than other areas of the wall (**Figure 9-9**).

Body Position

Whenever possible, choose cover that permits you to stand. If you are trapped for a long time, standing is the most comfortable and versatile position. You can shift your body slightly without exposing yourself and change your location quickly when the need arises.

If you cannot stand because of the height of the cover or the position of the assailant, squat rather than sit, and sit rather than lie. It is very difficult to change your position or location safely and swiftly from a prone position.

Changing Locations

Change locations only if the new location is better cover, farther from the hostile atmosphere, and can be reached without your revealing yourself to the assailant. Do not change your position of cover just for the sake of changing. Before changing locations, quickly look out from your cover several times (**Figure 9-10 A-C**). Look from a different height and angle each time. Use this "quick-peek" technique to evaluate the advisability of changing locations. Always return to cover as quickly as possible.

If you decide that you would be safer in another location, do not run directly away from the assailant's position; run in a zigzag pattern. You have less chance of being hit if your movement takes you across the assailant's field of view.

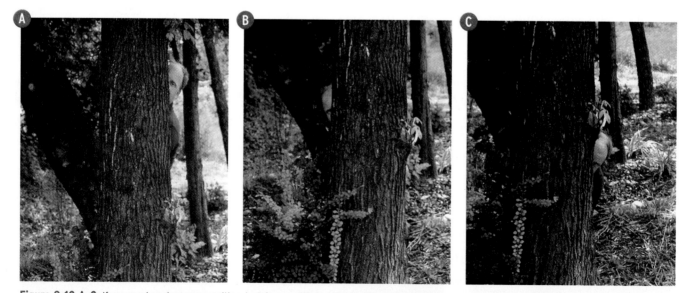

Figure 9-10 A-C If you must analyze your position, look from a different height and angle each time.

Concealment

Tall grass, shrubbery, and dark shadows are considered areas of concealment. When cover is not readily available, use concealment to provide some protection while you assess your position and seek cover.

Areas of concealment are more common after dark than during daylight hours. If you are involved in a violent situation at night, move into the darkness or shadows and stand still. The assailant cannot see you and may not shoot. If the assailant fires shots at random, chances are you will not be hit.

In rural areas, tall grass or a cornfield can conceal you whether it is day or night (**Figure 9-11**). Remain motionless so that the foliage does not move. After you finish analyzing the situation, move toward cover.

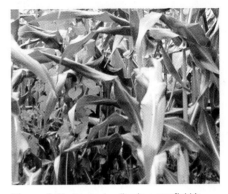

Figure 9-11 A man standing in a cornfield is practically invisible.

SURVIVAL TIPS

1) Unless you *know* the thickness and quality of material used in the construction of interior walls and furnishings, treat them as concealment, not cover.

2) Remember that when you are concealed, you cannot be seen by your assailant, but you can be heard. Move as quietly as possible.

3) If you are concealed from view behind a large bush or in a dark shadow, you may feel secure, but if a streetlight is behind you or an approaching vehicle silhouettes you in the headlights, you are again visible (**Figure 9-12**).

4) Do not look out from your cover to see what is happening. Until the area is secured, remain completely concealed from the assailant until you hear an all-clear.

5) Before you use darkness as concealment, remove all clothing with reflective tape. In cold temperatures or inclement weather, wear the garments inside out to protect you from the elements (**Figure 9-13**).

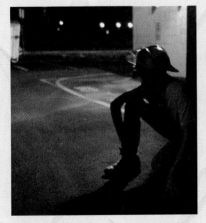

Figure 9-12 Do not stand between a light and your assailant.

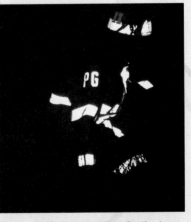

Figure 9-13 If not for the reflective tape, this firefighter would be invisible.

Chapter 10

Hostage Situations

On May 28, 1982, in Montgomery County, Maryland, a man crashed his car through the north entrance of the IBM building and ran through the building, randomly firing a machine gun at occupants. Firefighters and paramedics, armed only with their jump kits and good intentions, arrived before SWAT personnel and immediately entered the building without waiting for a safety clearance. When SWAT personnel, equipped with flak vests, M-16s, and tear gas, arrived and the fire chief was told about the nature of the incident, all fire department personnel (except the SWAT medics) were withdrawn from the building until it was secured and the area declared safe. By the end of the 7-hour incident, approximately 200 people had been treated or undergone triage and three had died (**Figure 10-1**).

Fire and EMS personnel sometimes arrive on a scene before it is secure. When law enforcement personnel arrive, they may try to include paramedics as members of the initial entry team.[1] If you have not been trained for this type of operation, do not participate in an assault on the aggressor's

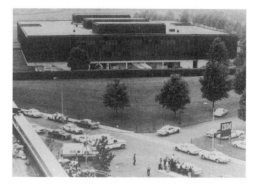

Figure 10-1 Police and rescue workers assembled outside IBM building. *(Courtesy Wide World Photos, NY)*

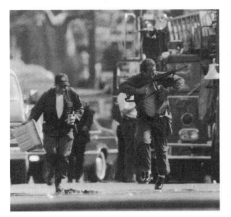

Figure 10-2 Fire department personnel remain in a secure staging area as law enforcement personnel change positions. *(Courtesy The Philadelphia Inquirer, Philadelphia, PA)*

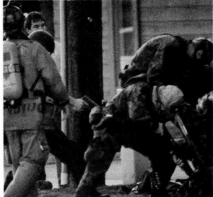

Figure 10-3 Fire, rescue, and EMS personnel must remain behind the police-barricade line until the area is secure. Would you consider this area secure? *(Courtesy Union-Tribune Publishing Co, San Diego, CA)*

position (**Figure 10-2**); you could be injured or taken hostage. Hostage situations are law enforcement problems until the scene is secure (**Figure 10-3**).

Surviving as a Hostage

Have you considered what you would do if you met an armed adversary? No rules apply; anything can happen depending on the assailant, your position, and your reactions.

The possibility of being taken hostage is extremely remote, but it does exist. If you are taken hostage, remember that most hostage incidents in the United States last between 4½ and 5 hours. Also remember that your behavior can greatly enhance your chances of surviving the ordeal.

Hostages are usually held as a form of human collateral to ensure compliance with a promise made by a person in authority. If you are taken hostage, you can increase your chances of survival if you can anticipate the feelings and actions of both the hostage taker and the negotiators. Statistics indicate that you have a 95% chance of surviving physically unharmed, if you remain calm (Hogewood W: Beltsville, MD, Prince Georges County Police Department, Special Operations Division, unpublished material on hostage taking, 1988).

The psychological problems that can develop are of greater concern than the possible physical abuse. Even if you are physically unharmed, you may experience some psychological problems during, and especially after, the incident. You may need professional counseling after the release to prevent long-term problems later. If you know what to expect as a hostage, you may have fewer psychological problems during the situation and after your release.

People Who Take Hostages

Hostage takers are generally classified as *crazies, criminals,* or *crusaders*.

Crazies. People who are mentally disturbed are involved in 52% of all hostage incidents.[2] A spouse, children, other relatives, or friends may be taken hostage. The mentally disturbed are rarely predictable and usually operate by a set of rules known only to themselves. Their reasons for taking hostages may be real or imagined. According to the FBI, these people typically fall into one of these diagnostic categories: paranoid schizophrenic, manic-depressive illness (depressed type), antisocial personality, or inadequate personality.[3]

Criminals. Criminals will take hostages to gain freedom from an unexpected entrapment. The hostages are usually people who are at the scene of the crime when something goes wrong, as in the following situation:

You stop the medic unit at a local convenience store to buy ice cream. The driver remains with the unit, and you enter the store and find a robbery in progress. The robber sees your uniform and the light bar on top of the unit and instantly panics. In his eyes, you are a cop—and he is in big trouble. You are suddenly taken hostage along with everyone else in the store.

Crusaders. Crusaders use the tactics of terror to attempt to further their cause. These groups can operate in any area, and their presence continues to grow. Extreme left-wing, right-wing, radical-religious, single-issue, or hate groups are found throughout the nation. Organizations such as the Ku Klux Klan, the United Freedom Front, the Armed Resistance Unit, and the May 19 Organization operate within the borders of the United States. As the events of September 11 have shown, terrorist groups from around the world can import violence into the United States.

The activities of international terrorists are well planned and precisely executed. You may become inadvertently involved in a terrorist action. If government offices, military installations, nuclear power plants, defense contractors, research facilities, or dams are in your area, you are susceptible to the threat. According to the International Association of Chiefs of Police (1978), only if you are completely familiar with and prepared for a confrontation with terrorism will you be equipped to survive with dignity.[4]

Stages of a Hostage Situation

The six stages involved in taking and maintaining hostages are outlined in the box *Six Stages of a Hostage Situation*. Emergency services workers who are taken hostage are most affected by the capture, transport, and holding stages.

Capture Stage. When an emergency services worker is taken hostage, the hostage taker is usually as surprised as the captured worker. Mentally disturbed individuals and criminals rarely plan to capture an emergency services worker, but if it happens, they may use the hostage as a medium of exchange or as a safety shield when they attempt to escape.[5]

During the capture, the hostage taker will probably be extremely nervous and trying to gain control of what has suddenly become an unsettled situation. At this stage, you are in grave personal danger. Assume that the person on the other end of the gun will use violence if you do not follow instructions.

Do not attempt to escape. Consider the safety of any other hostages. If your escape attempt fails, what will your new position be with your abductor? If your actions antagonize your captor, your chances of being hurt increase. You must avoid personal injury, remain calm, and control the instinctive anger that occurs when you are physically abused.

At the moment of capture, you may feel that it is all a bad dream because your mind cannot adjust quickly to such a radical change. The automatic defense of denial facilitates the transition from being in control of your surroundings to acknowledging your inability to defend yourself.[6]

Transport Stage. The hostage taker may order you to move to a more secure location. This move may be only to the other side of the room or to another part of the same building.

If you are transported soon after capture, the aggressor will still be agitated. During this stage, expect to receive harsh commands from your captor. If the captor feels you are moving too slowly, expect physical abuse such as pushing, dragging, or kicking.

If your abductor has time, you may be tied, gagged, and blindfolded before being transported. Your body may slip into shock, and if you

---

Box 10-1:   **Six Stages of a Hostage Situation**

Stage 1 – Surveillance. The terrorist group identifies and watches the intended hostage until they know the person's every move. Terrorists learn as much about the intended hostage as possible before making the capture.

Stage 2 – Capture. The hostage takers are usually excited, armed, and capable of violent actions.

Stage 3 – Transport. The terrorist group moves the hostage to a different location within the same general area, such as from behind the counter to the back storage.

Stage 4 – Holding. Negotiations begin for release of the hostage; the strain of waiting may affect the hostage psychologically.

Stage 5 – Move. The hostage is transported to an entirely different location than the site of capture.

Stage 6 – Resolution. The hostage is released after successful negotiations or an assault on the hostage taker's position by SWAT members.

have been slow in following instructions, you will experience physical pain and emotional instability. Your perceptions may be distorted, especially if you are blindfolded.

If you are prepared and have planned ahead, you can reduce the shock of this experience, recover your senses quickly, and regain your composure. Collect as much information as possible about your location by using all your senses, especially if you are blindfolded during the move. What do you hear? Are church bells ringing? Do you hear trains, airplanes, or street traffic? Are people talking in a foreign language? Do you smell animals, chemicals, or food? If you used stairs, try to remember the number of floors. Did you leave the original building? If you are transported by vehicle, analyze the route of travel. Count the number, the direction, and the order of turns. Be aware of outside noises that will help reconstruct the route. Note the number of captors involved and the types and quantity of weapons. The more you can remember about the transport stage of your captivity, the more help you will be to law enforcement agencies after your release.

Holding Stage. During the holding stage, many hostages may begin to develop psychological and emotional problems. The situation has calmed slightly, and law enforcement is at the scene and release negotiations are ongoing. The holding stage is tedious; you sit, wait, and hope for a safe release. Hostage negotiators count on time to bring an incident to a safe and successful conclusion. Your chances of survival increase proportionally from the time of your capture to the time of your release.[7] In the beginning stages, the hostage taker may threaten to kill you. But as time goes on, you are kept alive so that the hostage taker's demands will be met (**Figure 10-4**).

Even if negotiations have started, do not try predict an exact time or date of release, even to yourself. If you set an unrealistic goal (such as 4 hours) and are wrong, you will feel demoralized. Only your abductors will decide when or whether you will be released. If you have been captured by terrorists, plan for a much longer time in captivity than if your captors were criminals or mentally disturbed individuals. Accept the fact that you have no control over when you will be freed.

During the holding stage your mental state is a greater danger to you than your captors are. After you reach the holding area, your captors

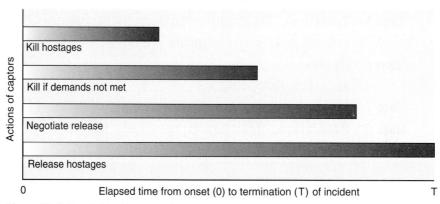

Figure 10-4 Thresholds of hostage safety.

will try to break your spirit. You may be forced to ask for food and permission to sleep or to use the toilet.[8]

Manage yourself and your personal environment. Do not do anything that will attract unwanted attention, and do not stare at your captors. If you convincingly fake a heart attack or sickness, you become less valuable and more expendable to your captors. If the hostage takers feel you are in their way or on their nerves, they may kill you. Remember that any one of your captors can walk in and kill you at any time. Your only chance for survival is in your role as a bargaining chip. Do not pressure or agitate them into changing their plans. Be especially careful of female hostage takers. They may get angry easily and turn to violence.

Hostage negotiators suggest you find a middle ground between being too daring and being a coward. A behavior continuum model (**Figure 10-5**) illustrates the danger zones and caution areas of your actions.

Because you are wearing a uniform, other hostages may look to you for guidance and strength. Your captors may consider this image of authority as a threat. Anything that draws attention to you increases the possibility of violence. Make every effort to be inconspicuous. Develop a nonthreatening image by removing the badge, collar pins, and patches from your uniform, or turn your uniform shirt inside out so these items are not visible.

Sometimes, when it comes to sanitary conditions or personal cleanliness, you will have to ignore normal definitions of modesty. Take advantage of the opportunity to bathe or use bathroom facilities, regardless of the presence of male or female guards or other hostages.

You may receive only one meal a day. When you are given food, divide it into three portions for breakfast, lunch, and supper. Try to maintain a normal, daily routine.

As your time in captivity increases, exercise becomes increasingly important to your physical and mental conditioning. Many soldiers who survived imprisonment during war continued to exercise, even when they were confined to a small box. This became a contributing factor to their survival.

Keeping your mind active is as important as exercising your body. Write letters (even if they will not be mailed), read anything you can find, and fantasize. Mental activity will help time pass more easily under adverse conditions.

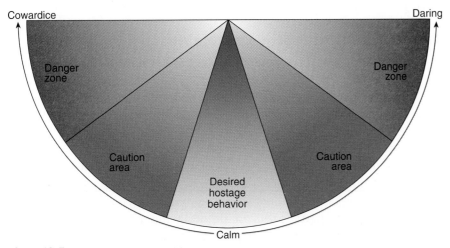

Figure 10-5 Behavior continuum model.

Measure time by the meals, the guard's behavior (for example, sleepy at night), and outside noises (birds in the morning, crickets at night). Keep a calendar of days and celebrate special events such as holidays and birthdays. Establish a daily routine for meals, personal hygiene, housekeeping your own space, rest, exercise, and sleeping periods.

The Stockholm Syndrome

The Stockholm Syndrome reflects an experience that long-term hostages may have. When both captors and hostages share the same experiences for more than three days, the hostages may begin to identify and bond with their captors more than the police and the outside world.

Identifying and bonding with captors is a psychological reaction to circumstances that force you to mentally fight for your life. Even if your life is threatened by your abductors, your survival instinct tells you that your captors must think of you as a friendly and cooperative person so that they will see you as empathic and spare your life. Because the captors spare your life, you may feel grateful to them and begin to look at them in a more sympathetic light.

The Stockholm Syndrome also affects the hostage taker. A captor who becomes friendly with hostages will not readily harm or kill them. After the hostage taker interacts with the hostages, the possibility of aggressive action against the hostages is reduced. Terrorist organizations know the danger of this happening and will frequently change guards over the hostages. To prevent human contact between guards and hostages, some organizations require guards to wear hoods to negate the effect of face-to-face contact.

For the Stockholm Syndrome to develop, there must be positive contacts between the hostages and the hostage takers. Humane actions by the hostage takers, such as allowing the hostages to use toilet facilities, giving them blankets when it is cold, or talking with them on a personal level, are signs that a relationship is beginning. The hostages will start to look at their captors as humans with problems similar to their own and may blame law enforcement personnel for their continued imprisonment. If the hostage takers subject the hostages to beatings, pain, dehumanizing living conditions, or other forms of negative association during their time in captivity, the syndrome will not develop.[9]

Law Enforcement Procedures in a Hostage Situation

Most modern law enforcement agencies either have or have access to a highly trained negotiating team. The number of members assigned to the team, the agencies represented, and the professional background of team members vary by jurisdiction. The one goal they all share is that the safety of the hostages comes first.

Until the negotiating team arrives on the scene, there may be no contact between law enforcement personnel and the hostage takers. Law enforcement officers recognize the value of time in a hostage situation. At the beginning of an incident involving hostages, emotions are usually high, and all of the participants are thinking and acting emotionally rather than rationally.[10] As time passes, the situation becomes less tense for all persons involved, including the police.

Whenever possible, negotiators should not attempt any contact with the hostage takers until the incident seems stabilized. The negotiators gather information about the hostages and the hostage takers during this waiting period. The negotiators will probably be talking with the abductors by telephone instead of face to face. The telephone ensures a private conversation and the safety of the negotiating parties.

Remember, after all demands for release or surrender have been met, the hostage takers will probably not escape successfully. If you are a hostage, stay away from doors and windows. After your captors have surrendered to the police or tried to escape, stay where you are. Do not leave the area where you were being held until you are told to do so by law enforcement personnel. If the police assault on your location in an attempted rescue, lie on the floor and place your hands on your head. Remain in that position until your rescuers tell you to move.

The time immediately after your rescue is just as critical to your safety as when you were first captured. The rescuers may not recognize you as a hostage and treat everyone in the room as a suspect. You must control your emotions and follow the rescuer's instructions completely. After you have been properly identified and the area is declared safe, you will have time to thank your rescuers.

SURVIVAL TIPS

1. Maintain your composure and remain calm.

2. Follow your captor's instructions completely.

3. Inform your captors of any medical problems. If you require scheduled medication, you may be released.

4. Do not stare at your captors. Be as inconspicuous as possible and do not make any sudden moves.

5. Accept the fact that you are a hostage. When you talk with your captors, do not antagonize them—talk in your normal voice.

6. Do not fight sleep. Resting is one way of reducing anxiety.

7. Accept any favors offered by your abductors, including food, beverages, and toilet privileges.

8. Do not try to overpower your captors. If you fail, the reaction against you may be violent and possibly fatal.

9. Stay clear of doors and windows. If law enforcement personnel assault the position, lie flat on the floor and remain motionless until you are instructed to move.

10. To prevent lasting emotional trauma, accept psychological counseling after a hostage experience.

11

Bombs, Booby Traps, and Makeshift Weapons

During the 1990s, there were a number of catastrophic bombing incidents in the United States. The 1993 bombing of the World Trade Center in New York killed six, injured 1,042, and caused $510 million in damage. The bombing of the Murrah Federal Building in Oklahoma City in 1995 took the lives of 168 innocent people, injured 518 people and caused $100 million in damage. As in the case of Theodore Kaczynski, some bombers are able to elude police for years. Kaczynski, known as the "Unabomber" killed three people and injured 22 others with 16 package bombs over a period of 18 years. Eric Rudolph, recently indicted for the Olympic Park bombing during the 1996 Olympic Games in Atlanta, also has eluded an intensive law enforcement manhunt for years.

The possibility that you, as an emergency responder, would encounter an explosive device, booby trap, or other makeshift weapon continues to increase. If you assume that a harmless-looking package, a normally safe area, or a calm, friendly individual will not present a threat, you invite disaster. Your attention to the possibility of violence should be peaked whenever you are on the street.

Box 11-1:   A Close Call

On April 29, 1997, Los Angeles County Fire Department units were dispatched to a female spotted over the side of a 300' cliff along the Pacific coastline. The first units on the scene found an unconscious female alone on a rocky beach—providing no information as to exactly what had occurred.

Some articles of clothing and a small cooler were found near the patient. As paramedics began to treat the patient, the cooler was moved to make room for a back-board. While the paramedics were treating the patient, fire-fighters spotted a loaded handgun and open cans of black powder in the vicinity.

Additional personnel arriving on scene from an air-rescue helicopter noted that there were wires coming from the cooler that had been moved moments earlier. Believing that the cooler could contain an explosive device, the woman was quickly moved a safe distance from the device.

Treatment continued at the scene as the patient's condition deteriorated. She eventually went into cardiac arrest and was rushed to the hospital. At the emergency department, a surprised staff found a loaded and cocked derringer pistol in the back pocket of the patient's pants.

Back at the beach where the patient was first found, the bomb squad personnel from Los Angeles County Sheriff's Department arrived and appraised the situation. They finally detonated the device in the cooler at the scene. A powerful explosion resulted. No emergency medical personnel were harmed. What began as a routine call could have been deadly.

Who Uses Explosives?

Explosives are used in many civilian and military occupations. For example, companies that build roads, demolish buildings, and perform mining operations use explosives on a daily basis. When used legally, explosives are employed by well-trained professionals to accomplish a task. However, each year hundreds of pounds of explosives are stolen from private industry and the military. Over 50,000 pounds of explosives and 30,000 detonators were reported stolen throughout the United States between 1993 and 1997.[1]

Exercise caution whenever you respond to a location where explosives may be used. In one case, Kansas City firefighters were battling a pick-up truck fire on a construction site. When they saw smoke also coming from a nearby trailer, they proceeded to investigate. Six fire-fighters were killed when 45,000 pounds of ammonium nitrate, contained in that and an adjoining trailer, exploded.

A variety of groups and individuals may use explosives illegally to further a cause, intimidate a former spouse, or just experiment with a recipe found in a book or on the Internet. The person or group may be attempting to gain quick recognition, take revenge, or simply get some thrills.

Illegal drug users may protect their operations by using booby traps. Even normally law-abiding citizens such as small-business owners may install illegal booby traps to protect their property. Remember that anyone can use a makeshift weapon, whether it is an umbrella used in anger or a carefully constructed pipe bomb used with the intent to kill.

Bombs and Explosives

The number of bombing incidents in recent years has increased drastically. According to the FBI's Bomb Data Center, there were 848 bombing incidents in 1987. In 1994, there were 3,163. Between 1987 and 1997, there were 23,613 bombing incidents. In these incidents, 448 people died and 4,170 were injured.[2] These numbers underscore how important it is for emergency services personnel to become familiar with different kinds of explosives.

Explosives are generally classified as *low explosives*, *primary high explosives*, or *secondary high explosives*. Low explosives include black powder and rifle powder. They are readily available and are usually preferred by those with little experience or knowledge of explosives (**Figure 11-1**). Low explosives burn suddenly and violently at speeds up to 3,300 feet per second and produce pressures of approximately 30,000 pounds per square inch (psi).[3]

Primers and detonators are the two major types of primary high explosives. Blasting caps, which are used to detonate the main explosive charge, are initiated with an electrical signal or a burning time fuse (**Figure 11-2**). Blasting caps are extremely sensitive to heat, shock, and friction, and their distribution is under tight control. However, caps

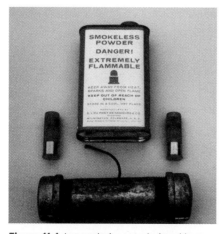

Figure 11-1 Low explosives are designed to propel bullets, but when confined in a pipe bomb, they can be deadly.

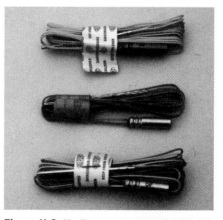

Figure 11-2 Blasting caps are approximately ¼" in diameter and 1" to 6" long. A copper or aluminum case is closed at one end and contains a measured amount of primary high explosive.

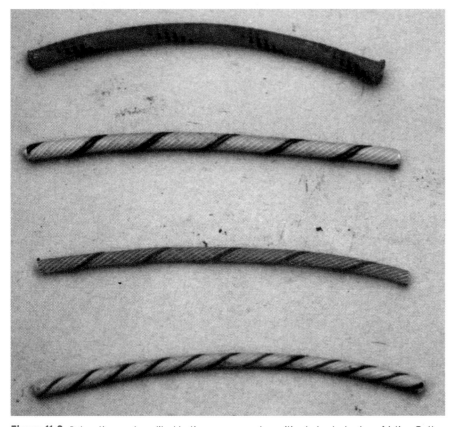

Figure 11-3 Detonating cords, unlike blasting caps, are not sensitive to heat, shock, or friction. To the uninformed emergency responder this may appear to be rescue rope.

may be stolen from construction sites and authorized storage areas for illegal use.[4]

Detonating cords, or Detcords, or Primacords, are used to transmit the detonating wave from the initiating source to the main charge. They are strong, flexible cords with a ¼" diameter and a center core containing primary high explosives (**Figure 11-3**). Properly trained individuals can use Detcords or Primacords to produce significant damage.

Secondary high explosives (such as dynamite and TNT) are relatively insensitive to heat, shock, and friction (**Figure 11-4**). Small, unconfined

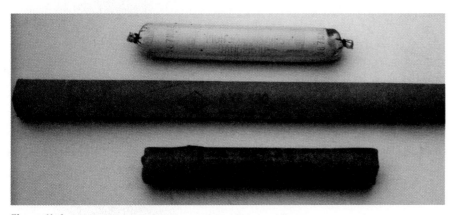

Figure 11-4 Secondary high explosives may appear to be road flares.

quantities of these explosives will usually burn instead of exploding when exposed to fire. However, when detonated, they produce as much as 1 million psi of pressure and can travel at speeds of 1,000 miles per second (m/s) to 8,500 m/s.[5]

Emergency personnel at the scene of a confirmed incident involving explosives or a reported bomb scare must have a working knowledge of proper operating procedures. Jurisdictions that have control over incidents involving bombs or other explosives need to develop protocols for a reported or suspected bomb, for a confirmed explosive device, and for postexplosion operations. Emergency personnel must not participate in any incident involving explosives until they have been thoroughly trained and are properly equipped and protected. If you are not, stop the operation. After all prerequisites have been met, continue the operation with extreme caution.

Preparation and Preplanning

With the threat of terrorism in the United States, many jurisdictions are reevaluating their response to bombing incidents. Some departments are now training their hazardous materials units to assist bomb squads in disposing of suspected improvised explosive devices. If the device contains a chemical or biological agent, trained personnel for such an eventuality will be in close proximity. In response to this new threat, many bomb squad members are also becoming certified as HazMat specialists or technicians.

Joint training sessions should be conducted with those agencies responsible for handling such incidents in your response district. These may include: local and state police; the FBI; the Bureau of Alcohol, Tobacco and Firearms, and military explosive ordinance disposal units. Develop policies and procedures that designate each agency's responsibility. This will alleviate confusion on the scene. Training sessions should include practicing the procedures for removing bomb suits. These suits are cumbersome. Emergency responders should not wait for an incident in their community to ask for details on suit removal.

Responders must also become familiar with the types of injuries that result from an explosion and their treatment. Consult your local protocols on how to treat primary, secondary, and tertiary blast injuries.

Each jurisdiction should conduct a community assessment to identify any potential targets that might appeal to a bomber or terrorist. The assessment should be a joint effort among law enforcement, fire, and EMS. Consider all government offices as targets. A person whose property tax assessment doubled may attempt to place an explosive device in the local courthouse. Perhaps a person who was denied a building permit wants to teach a lesson to the bureaucrats in the planning office. Family planning, abortion providers, and women's health clinics are also prime targets. If the clinic is located in the local hospital complex, there would be area-wide ramifications. A laboratory that does animal testing may be the target of an animal right's group.

Many departments link target hazard information from prefire planning to their dispatch computers. Information from the community assessment should also be linked to dispatch computers as a "threat hazard." This will then alert units responding to a given address, whether they be law enforcement or fire or rescue personnel, about the potential for problems.

Reported or Suspected Bomb in the Area

When you arrive on the scene of a bomb scare or suspicious package with a possible explosive, locate a knowledgeable representative from the area. This may be a family member if the incident is at a residence or a business representative if it occurs at a commercial or industrial establishment.

A form developed by the FBI contains pertinent questions to ask and information to gather during a bomb threat (**Figure 11-5**). This informa-

A

FBI
BOMB DATA CENTER

Place This Card Under Your Telephone

QUESTIONS TO ASK:

1. When is the bomb going to explode?

2. Where is it right now?

3. What does it look like?

4. What kind of bomb is it?

5. What will cause it to explode?

6. Did you place the bomb?

7. Why?

8. What is your address?

9. What is your name?

EXACT WORDING OF THE THREAT:

_____

_____

_____

_____

_____

_____

Sex of caller: _____ Race: _____
Age: _____ Length of call: _____

Number at which call is received:

_____

Time: _____ Date: ___ / ___ / ___

BOMB THREAT

FBI/DOJ

B

CALLER'S VOICE:

___ Calm		___ Nasal	
___ Angry		___ Stutter	
___ Excited		___ Lisp	
___ Slow		___ Raspy	
___ Rapid		___ Deep	
___ Soft		___ Ragged	
___ Loud		___ Clearing throat	
___ Laughter		___ Deep breathing	
___ Crying		___ Cracking voice	
___ Normal		___ Disguised	
___ Distinct		___ Accent	
___ Slurred		___ Familiar	
	___ Whispered		

If voice is familiar, who did it sound like?

_____

_____

BACKGROUND SOUNDS:

___ Street noises	___ Factory machinery	
___ Crockery	___ Animal noises	
___ Voices	___ Clear	
___ PA System	___ Static	
___ Music	___ Local	
___ House noises	___ Long distance	
___ Motor	___ Booth	
___ Office machinery	Other _____	

THREAT LANGUAGE:

___ Well spoken (educated)	___ Incoherent
___ Foul	___ Taped
___ Irrational	___ Message read by threat maker

REMARKS: _____

_____

_____

Report call immediately to:

_____

Phone number _____

Date ___ / ___ / ___

Name _____

Position _____

Phone number _____

Figure 11-5 These or similar cards should be distributed to all business and government offices.

tion is critical in assessing the credibility of the threat. A similar card should be distributed throughout the local business and government community. Unfortunately, most serious bombers rarely phone-in a threat to their targets.[6]

Any information obtained by the person who takes the call will be useful. The expected time of detonation and the location of the device are the most important questions you should ask. If time permits, obtain floor plans of the building and make enough copies on a copy machine in a nearby building so that each search team has plans of its assigned search areas. Fire department prefire plans may also prove useful.

Before you issue an evacuation order, have the occupants examine the immediate area around them for anything suspicious. These individuals will have the greatest knowledge of their surroundings and will be able to spot an abnormal object. Instruct them not to touch anything suspicious, but to report their findings to on-scene emergency responders, who should then communicate the information to the incident commander. To keep panic to a minimum, officials may elect to quietly evacuate the building, perhaps on the pretense of a fire alarm. In this case, only key individuals from the building would be used to search the premises. Evacuees should be kept a safe distance from the scene; the *2000 Emergency Response Guidebook* suggests a *minimum* of 330'[17] (**Figure 11-6**). On-scene law enforcement personnel can assist in determining a safe distance. Remember that the range of flying glass and debris from a bomb will be far greater than you might expect.

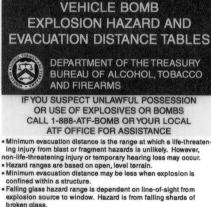

ATF	VEHICLE DESCRIPTION	MAXIMUM EXPLOSIVES CAPACITY	LETHAL AIR BLAST RANGE	MINIMUM EVACUATION DISTANCE	FALLING GLASS HAZARD
	COMPACT SEDAN	500 Pounds 227 Kilos *(In Trunk)*	100 Feet 30 Meters	1,500 Feet 457 Meters	1,250 Feet 381 Meters
	FULL SIZE SEDAN	1,000 Pounds 455 Kilos *(In Trunk)*	125 Feet 38 Meters	1,750 Feet 534 Meters	1,750 Feet 534 Meters
	PASSENGER VAN OR CARGO VAN	4,000 Pounds 1,818 Kilos	200 Feet 61 Meters	2,750 Feet 838 Meters	2,750 Feet 838 Meters
	SMALL BOX VAN (14 FT BOX)	10,000 Pounds 4,545 Kilos	300 Feet 91 Meters	3,750 Feet 1,143 Meters	3,750 Feet 1,143 Meters
	BOX VAN OR WATER/FUEL TRUCK	30,000 Pounds 13,636 Kilos	450 Feet 137 Meters	6,500 Feet 1,982 Meters	6,500 Feet 1,982 Meters
	SEMI-TRAILER	60,000 Pounds 27,273 Kilos	600 Feet 183 Meters	7,000 Feet 2,134 Meters	7,000 Feet 2,134 Meters

ATF I 5400.1 (01-99)

ATF

VEHICLE BOMB EXPLOSION HAZARD AND EVACUATION DISTANCE TABLES

DEPARTMENT OF THE TREASURY BUREAU OF ALCOHOL, TOBACCO AND FIREARMS

IF YOU SUSPECT UNLAWFUL POSSESSION OR USE OF EXPLOSIVES OR BOMBS CALL 1-888-ATF-BOMB OR YOUR LOCAL ATF OFFICE FOR ASSISTANCE

• Minimum evacuation distance is the range at which a life-threatening injury from blast or fragment hazards is unlikely. However, non-life-threatening injury or temporary hearing loss may occur.
• Hazard ranges are based on open, level terrain.
• Minimum evacuation distance may be less when explosion is confined within a structure.
• Falling glass hazard range is dependent on line-of-sight from explosion source to window. Hazard is from falling shards of broken glass.
• Metric equivalent values are mathematically calculated.
• Explosion confined within a structure may cause structural collapse or building debris hazards.
• Additional hazards include vehicle debris.

This information was developed with data from the Dipole Might vehicle bomb research program conducted by ATF, with technical assistance from the U.S. Army Corps of Engineers. Goals for Dipole Might include creating a computerized database and protocol for investigating large-scale vehicle bombs. Dipole Might is sponsored by the Technical Support Working Group (TSWG). TSWG is the research and development arm of the National Security Council interagency working group on counterterrorism.

ATF I 5400.1 (01-99)

Figure 11-6 The Bureau of Alcohol, Tobacco and Firearms provides information on minimum evacuation distances for a variety of vehicle bombs.

Conducting the Search

Properly trained and equipped personnel should conduct searches for suspicious packages that might contain explosive devices (**Figure 11-7**). Searches should be conducted room by room. Depending upon their size, rooms should be searched by two individuals. Begin the search by looking from the floor to waist height. Then check from waist height to eye level, and finally from eye level to the ceiling.[8] Give special consideration to void areas in rooms that have false ceilings. Search public areas such as hallways, restrooms, lobbies, stairwells, and auditoriums first. Do not handle or in any way disturb a suspicious item.

Confirmed Explosive Device

When you arrive on the scene of a confirmed explosive device, you should designate an initial command post and staging area for additional fire and EMS units. This area may be as far as 3,000' from the incident site, depending on the type of explosive device (US Department of Justice, Washington DC, unpublished material from a training program). The initial incident commander (IC) should meet with law enforcement personnel for a briefing on the situation. As with any emergency incident, the IC must then develop strategic goals and tactical objectives as well as an overall incident or mission plan (see Chapter 14). A unified command system between law enforcement and fire officials is the most appropriate for this type of operation.

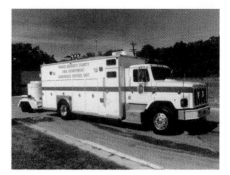

Figure 11-7 Hazardous Devices Unit, Prince Georges County Fire Department, MD.

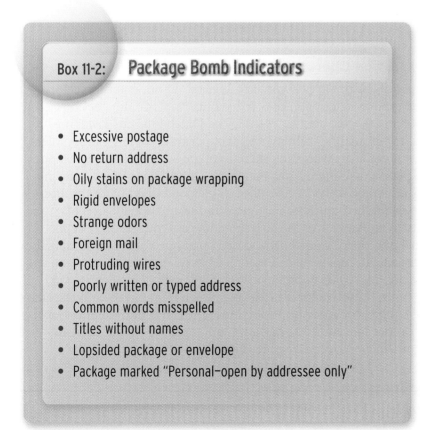

Box 11-2:   **Package Bomb Indicators**

- Excessive postage
- No return address
- Oily stains on package wrapping
- Rigid envelopes
- Strange odors
- Foreign mail
- Protruding wires
- Poorly written or typed address
- Common words misspelled
- Titles without names
- Lopsided package or envelope
- Package marked "Personal—open by addressee only"

If law enforcement intends to disarm the device, joint plans must be developed to address emergency actions in the event of a detonation. If untrained fire, rescue, or EMS personnel are in the danger zone when the device explodes, they become part of the problem instead of part of the solution. A forward staging area may be necessary in certain situations. For example, if the device is on the tenth floor of an office building, a small contingent of fire and EMS personnel may be staged two or three floors below. This allows for a quicker and safer response from within the structure. If all units are staged outside the structure, falling glass after a detonation may be hazardous to crews attempting to enter the building. Command officers should be guided by the wishes and experience of bomb squad personnel, who can more accurately determine a safe perimeter. This will be based upon, among other things, the size of the device.

Complicating these situations is the possibility of a second device, meant to injure or kill emergency response personnel. On January 16, 1997, an explosive device detonated in an abortion clinic in Fulton County, Georgia. Approximately one hour after the initial explosion, a second device exploded. Seven people, including a firefighter and an ATF agent, were injured. Little more than a month later, four people were injured when a gay nightclub in Atlanta was bombed. Investigators found a second device in a backpack on top of a wall. Emergency responders are being targeted by secondary devices.

You should assume that a second device is present. Always conduct an initial search around the command post, staging areas, and evacuation areas. Identify any out-of-place packages or objects and notify the IC. The unified command will announce and direct searches of other areas.

Postexplosion Operations

Because of the threat of secondary devices, do not enter the detonation area until it is declared safe. Triage must wait; do not commit personnel to an unstable area for rescue. The Oklahoma City bombing showed how structural stability may hamper rescue efforts. Responders must not enter areas where the stability of the structure is in question.

Each person entering the detonation area must be identified; remember, this is a crime scene. A controlled single point of entry for the area must be established quickly. Someone with the appropriate level of authority to limit access to the area should be assigned to this location. All personnel movement should be recorded on a sign-in sheet, including the name, the agency represented, a work telephone number, the time in, and the time out. Make this information part of the official incident report.

Take notes on your observations and actions. Do not disturb the area any more than absolutely necessary during rescue and firefighting operations. Do not move dead bodies until told to do so by the authority having jurisdiction over the scene (**Figure 11-8**).

Booby Traps

Booby traps have become a serious threat to emergency responders. These devices can be used as alarms for early warning or to maim and

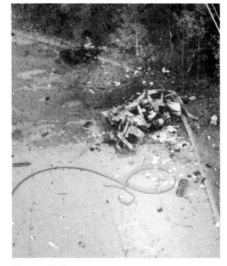

Figure 11-8 Emergency responders must be careful not to disturb evidence at a bombing incident. In this incident where a man killed himself and his family with an explosive device, evidence is scattered throughout a large area. *(Courtesy Baltimore County Police Department, Baltimore, MD)*

kill. Often, criminals will use booby traps to protect a marijuana-growing operation or a methamphetamine lab. Booby traps do not discriminate. The innocent civilian or the well-intentioned firefighter or emergency medical technician can fall victim to these devices.

An article in *Firehouse* magazine entitled "Firefighting Today" tells the sad truth, as these examples show. A drug dealer whose apartment has a fire escape running past his bedroom window fears that his product might be stolen. He wires the ladder with a live current and electrocutes the unknowing firefighter trying to "make the roof" via the fire escape. Or perhaps the dealer drives large nails through a piece of plywood or a 2" × 4" piece of lumber, and places it on the floor just inside the window (**Figure 11-9**). The firefighter attempting to enter the room can be severely injured as he steps on the nails. The nails or spikes may be coated with poisonous chemicals, possibly even fecal matter. Similar devices were called "punji stakes" during the conflict in Vietnam. Another booby trap might involve fish hooks hanging from the ceiling at eye level. In a dimly lighted room, they might not be seen and can do permanent damage to eyes. Fish hook booby traps have also been found along outdoor hiking paths leading to marijuana fields, hanging from trees, at eye level, on monofilament line. People have even turned normal warning systems, such as guard dogs, into booby traps. If the owner has the dog's voice box surgically removed, it can't bark. A paramedic responding to the apartment for an overdose may be unaware of trouble until the dog bites his leg.[9]

There are also chemical booby traps. A glass of hydrochloric acid may be placed behind the closed entry door to a house or apartment and positioned to tip into a plate filled with cyanide pellets when the door is opened. The mixture of the two chemicals produces hydrogen cyanide gas, which is used to execute prisoners in some penitentiaries. A more typical booby trap involves a light bulb filled with gasoline and placed in a light fixture. When some unsuspecting person turns on the light, the bulb explodes. A coffee can filled with acid and balanced on a partially opened door can cause painful burns to the unsuspecting responder who passes through the entryway.

Many homes have steel bars at the windows and doors. Such devices leave residents with a greater sense of security in high crime areas. But in their attempts to deter police during a raid, drug dealers have, on occasion, charged these bars with 220 volts of electricity.

Handgrenades are another popular device used in booby traps. A piece of monofilament line, virtually undetectable, can be strung across a path or doorway to act as a tripwire and detonate the grenade (**Figure 11-10**). Over 2,000 hand grenades were recovered by law enforcement in 1997.[10]

In one incident, firefighters were advised by police not to enter the residence where the fire was burning. This advice was based on the police department's past experience with the occupant. The firefighters controlled and extinguished the fire from outside the residence and then waited until the bomb squad arrived on the scene. The bomb squad found many booby traps throughout the house, including a hand grenade attached to the back door (the usual point of entry for an inte-

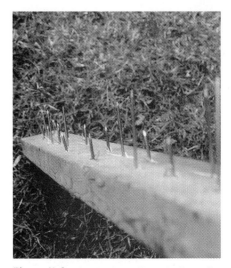

Figure 11-9 A two-by-four with protruding nails is used as a booby trap.

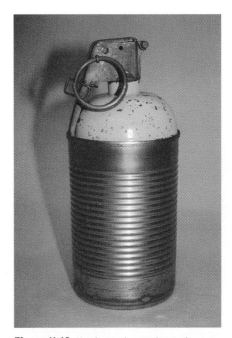

Figure 11-10 Handgrenades can be used as booby traps either outdoors or indoors. This grenade stuffed inside a soup can might be set atop a partially open door. As the door is opened the grenade falls from its perch and out of the can, exploding.

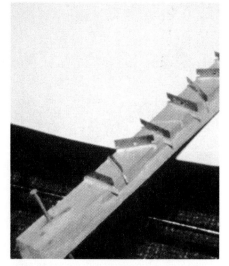

Figure 11-11 Board embedded with razor blades used to booby trap windows in a residence. *(Courtesy William S. Ennis, Sr., West Carrolton Division of Fire, West Carrollton, OH)*

rior attack on a fire in the front part of a house). The grenade was set to explode when the door was opened. Every window in the house had 1" × 2" strips of wood embedded with razor blades attached to the inside of the sill so that anyone who entered through the window would be severely injured (**Figure 11-11**).

Because the police arrived before the fire department and were familiar with the occupant, they were able to prevent injuries. If the fire department had arrived first and automatically followed normal procedures, the results would have been devastating.

A person who sets a deadly device may not intend to harm emergency personnel. But once the device is in place, there is no way to control who will be the victim. A careless step or gesture may lead to death or serious injury. If you find a possible booby trap, note its location and retreat to a safe location. Call for police and the bomb squad. If a member of your crew is injured by a booby trap, do not immediately rush to his aid. There may be a secondary device. Only the closest team member should carefully approach the injured person and evacuate to safety.

When you treat a patient in questionable surroundings, be careful what you touch, pick up, or move. Normal-looking household items are often used to rig booby traps.

Makeshift Weapons

Weapons come in many shapes and sizes; those that are the most deadly may not even look like weapons. After a weapon is activated, it is usually too late to avoid an injury. The harmless-looking fountain pen shown in **Figure 11-12 A**, can become a deadly weapon. When the shirt clip is depressed, it expels a spring-loaded, sharp rod from the end of the pen (**Figure 11-12 B**).

Many weapons are designed to be concealed under articles of clothing or disguised to look like harmless accessories. When the key ring shown in **Figure 11-13 A,** is unscrewed, it becomes a knife (**Figure 11-13 B**).

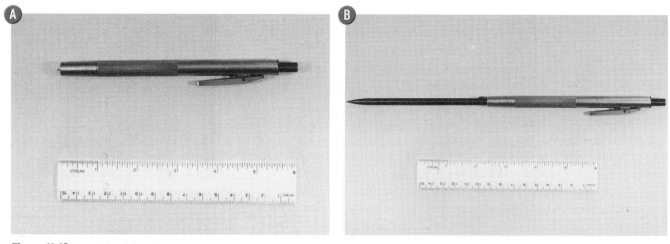

Figure 11-12   A. A 6" fountain pen?   **B.** Or a deadly weapon?

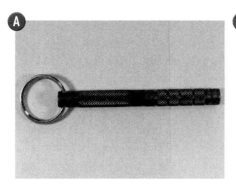

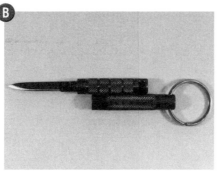

Figure 11-13 **A.** A harmless, 5" key ring?   **B.** Or a deadly weapon?

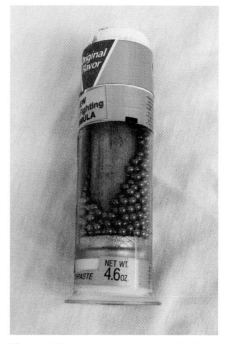

Figure 11-14 A toothpaste container with BBs that, when packed around a pipe bomb, become shrapnel when the device detonates.

Explosives can be concealed in many innocent-looking products. **Figure 11-14** shows a pipe bomb inside a toothpaste container. The cigarette lighter in **Figure 11-15** is an antipersonnel weapon designed to hold explosives. After the fuse is lit, the device is thrown at the intended victim. The explosion turns the metal container into shrapnel. **Figure 11-16** shows a small motion detector attached to an explosive device. Once the device is armed, any movement by an individual triggers an explosion. The motion detector is available from any corner electronics store for less than $15.

The key ring in **Figure 11-17** looks similar to the lavatory key rings used at many gas stations. A large object is attached to the lavatory key so that it will not be easily lost. This object, however, is known as a "ninja key ring." Intended for hand-to-hand combat, it is available at any martial arts supply store for under $5. When it is held in a closed fist, the shorter metal rods protrude past the fingers. The rods are placed so that a blow to the face results in piercing the victim's eyes. The longer metal bar protruding from the closed fist is capable of penetrating a person's skull.

When transporting patients from correctional facilities and police stations, thoroughly search them for weapons before you leave. Your search may reveal something as innocent looking as a bar of soap in a

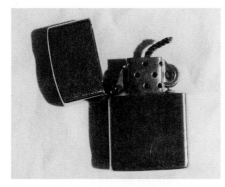

Figure 11-15 With the addition of explosives and a fuse, a lighter becomes an antipersonnel weapon.

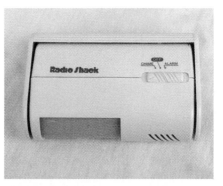

Figure 11-16 A cheap motion detector from the corner electronics store can be rigged to an explosive charge to form a sophisticated device.

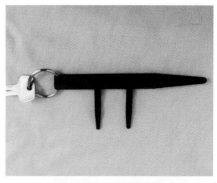

Figure 11-17 Use of the ninja key ring in hand-to-hand combat greatly improves attackers ability to permanently injure or kill their victim.

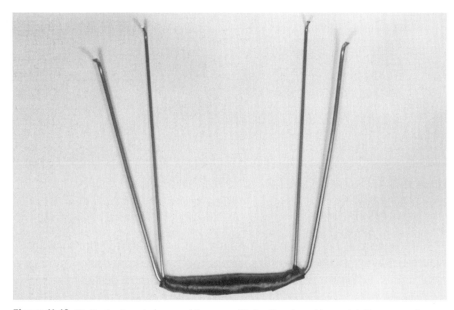

Figure 11-18 "Cat's claw" made from coat hangers with the tips shaved to a point. The weapon is hand-held and raked across the victim's face.

sock to a "cat's claw" (**Figure 11-18**). Request law enforcement personnel to conduct the search in your presence. If they refuse, complete a detailed survey of the patient and determine the number and extent of injuries before you accept the patient for transport.

When you are called to a scene involving a patient suspected of a violent crime, remove all of the patient's clothing while you conduct the survey and before you load the patient into the unit. This action will ensure that the patient is not armed.

Do not allow women to carry a purse on the stretcher. Weapons can easily be concealed in a purse (**Figure 11-19**). Place the purse on the squad bench where the patient can see it but cannot reach it.

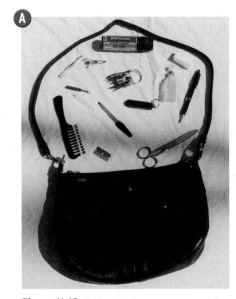

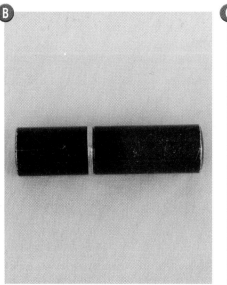

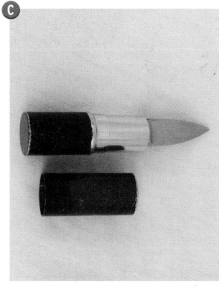

Figure 11-19 A. A women's purse can conceal an endless number of makeshift weapons.

B. An ordinary tube of lipstick.

C. Or is it?

Figures 11-20 through 11-35 show makeshift or concealed weapons. Study them and determine how you would react if you found one of these items on a patient you were treating.

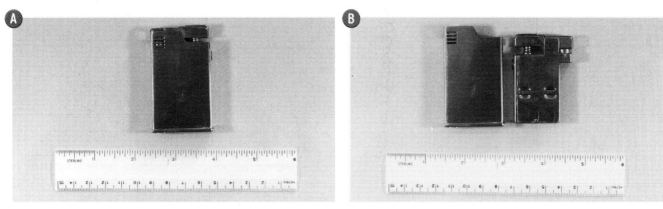

Figure 11-20 A. Cigarette lighter originally designed to fire small rounds of tear gas.

B. It has been altered to fire a .22-caliber round.

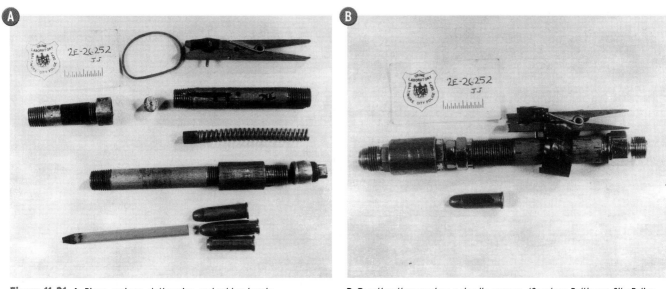

Figure 11-21 A. Pipes, springs, clothespins, and rubber bands.

B. Together they produce a deadly weapon. *(Courtesy Baltimore City Police Department, Baltimore, MD)*

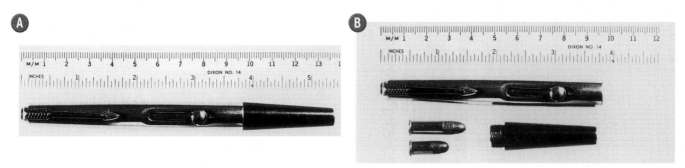

Figure 11-22 A. A normal-looking pen.

B. It fires a small-caliber round. *(Courtesy Baltimore City Police Department, Baltimore, MD)*

Figure 11-23 Another normal-looking pen. It opens to form a knife. *(Courtesy Baltimore City Police Department, Baltimore, MD)*

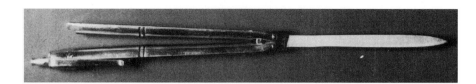

Figure 11-24 A .25-caliber semiautomatic handgun that can be concealed in the palm of the hand.

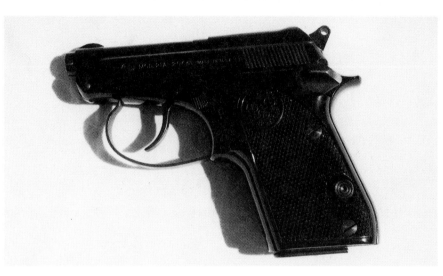

Figure 11-25 This small-caliber revolver can be concealed in the pager case. *(Courtesy Baltimore City Police Department, Baltimore, MD)*

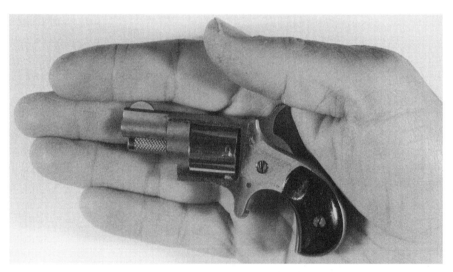

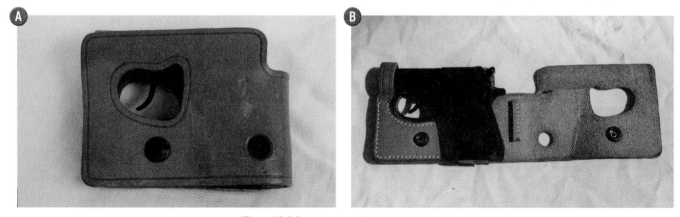

Figure 11-26 A. A man's wallet. **B.** It contains a .25-caliber semiautomatic weapon. Pistol can be fired without opening the wallet.

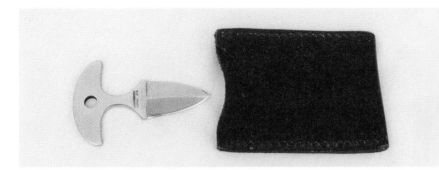

Figure 11-27 This wallet contains a push dagger.

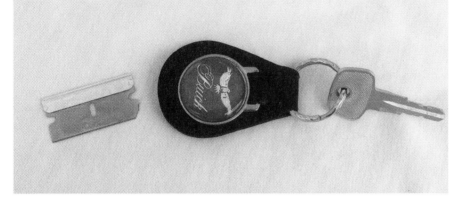

Figure 11-28 Razor blades and handcuff keys can be hidden in the leather tab of a key ring.

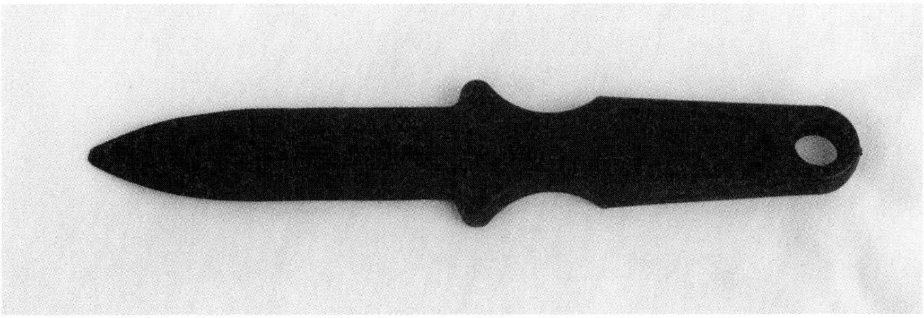

Figure 11-29 This knife made of a composite material will not be detected by a metal detector.

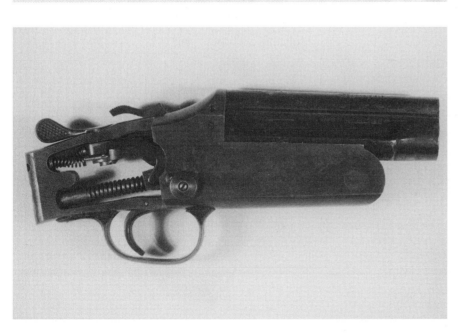

Figure 11-30 An easily concealed shotgun with the stock and most of the barrel removed. This weapon is not much larger than a man's hand.

Figure 11-31 Homemade guns of different calibers. Number five is a large firecracker wrapped with nails and tape. When the firecracker explodes, the nails become flying shrapnel. (*Courtesy Baltimore City Police Department, Baltimore, MD*)

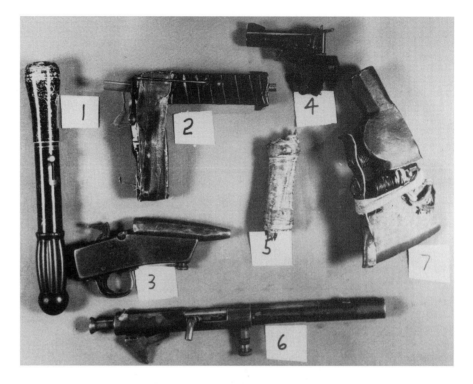

Figure 11-32 This 9-mm semiautomatic weapon is a favorite of drug dealers, it has a 35-round clip.

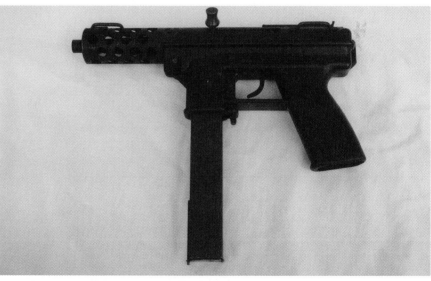

Figure 11-33 Known as a toe popper, this booby trap is planted in the ground. The device contains a shotgun shell. When an unsuspecting person steps on the buried device it acts like a land mine blowing the end of the person's foot off.

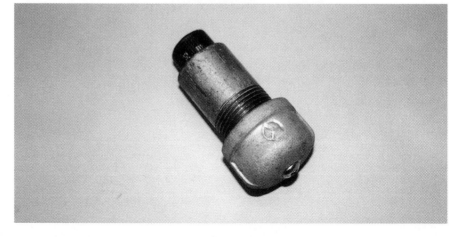

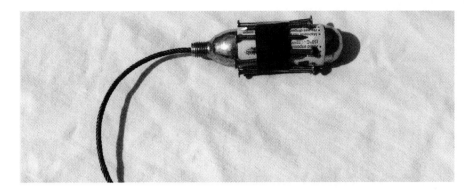

Figure 11-34 Known as a crickett, this explosive device is made from a CO_2 cartridge. Its lethality is increased by wrapping it with nails. Many of these devices were found at Columbine High School.

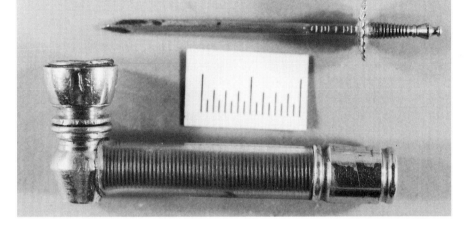

Figure 11-35 A crack pipe with hidden knife. *(Courtesy Baltimore County Police Department, Baltimore, MD)*

SURVIVAL TIPS

1 Bombers are leaving secondary explosives that target emergency responders and increase chaos.

2 Booby traps do not discriminate. Once they have been set, they can harm anyone in the area, even the person who set them.

3 Never assume that a patient will not attack you because you are trying to help. Identify and move any items that can be used as makeshift weapons out of the patient's reach.

4 If you find an unusual object, possibly a bomb or a booby trap, during your approach or patient care activities, withdraw to a safe area (taking the patient with you, if possible), and notify the proper authorities. Under no circumstances should anyone other than a trained bomb-disposal expert disturb the object.

5 If law enforcement personnel decide to inspect the object before calling the bomb squad, ask them to wait until you and your patient move a safe distance from the object.

6 It is better to have people laugh at you for being overcautious than to have them mourn you for being careless.

Chapter 12

Clandestine Drug Laboratories

As the war against drugs intensifies, more illegal drug manufacturing laboratories are established within the United States. The efforts of law enforcement agencies to limit illegal drug trafficking from other countries have forced many dealers and users to produce dangerous substances in clandestine labs. The volatile nature and toxic effects of the chemicals involved, as well as the unpredictable responses of drug users, increases the physical danger for emergency services personnel who may not realize the incident involves an illicit drug operation.

Several substances are abused for their mind-altering effects. Cocaine is made from coca plant, which is grown throughout South America. The opium poppy is grown widely in Asia and is used to make both morphine and heroin. Marijuana is grown throughout the world, including within the United States. Other substances are synthesized, including lysergic acid diethylamide (LSD), phencyclidine (PCP), and gamma-hydroxy-butyrate (GHB), and manufactured in clandestine labs. Today, the most popular manufactured substance is methamphetamine, known on the street as "meth," "speed," or "crank."

With a small investment of a few hundred dollars, a cooker (drug manufacturer) can begin producing pure methamphetamine. The necessary chemicals to produce just 1 ounce of the drug cost less than $100. But the street value will often exceed $1,800 (J Lofland, Intelligence Analyst, Drug Enforcement Administration, personal communication, 2001). Methamphetamine sales exceeded $3 billion in 1988, and production fell short of the 25-ton annual demand for the drug.[1]

The proliferation of illegal drug labs continues. In 1999, 2,155 methamphetamine labs were seized by the Drug Enforcement Administration (DEA),[2] and 7,528 lab seizures were reported by state and local agencies.[3] In the Midwest, where 90% of drug cases involve methamphetamine, the number of labs seized by law enforcement increased tenfold in just 2 years.[4] Labs are located in every state; even rural states like Kentucky reported 68 lab seizures in 1999.[5]

Location of Illegal Drug Laboratories

Clandestine drug laboratories are found in every geographic and socioeconomic area. They can be found in cheap inner-city hotels, in expensive suburban homes, and in small trailer camps throughout rural America. Labs are found in vehicles such as buses, trucks, and motor homes (**Figure 12-1 A-B**).

Recognizing Illegal Drug Laboratories

In general, there are two ways to produce methamphetamine. The first starts with a chemical known as phenyl-2-propanone (P-2-P). This method requires fairly sophisticated equipment and takes 24 to 36 hours to complete the chemical process that produces the drug. The second method is preferred not only because it is simpler, but also because it produces a drug that is two to three times more potent. In this method, ephedrine or pseudoephedrine is used as the basis for production.

The quality and quantity of equipment varies greatly. A basic laboratory may mix the compounds in buckets (**Figure 12-2**), but there are also elaborate laboratories that use sophisticated glassware, heating mantles, and vacuum equipment (**Figure 12-3**). Newer labs are virtually disposable. The cooker uses over-the-counter cold remedies containing ephedrine or pseudoephedrine. Approximately 400 to 600 pills are ground in a household blender, then combined with denatured alcohol

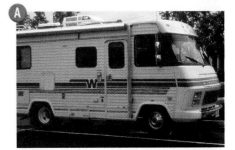

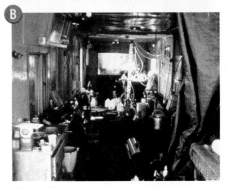

Figure 12-1 Motor homes are often used as mobile cooking labs. **A.** From the outside, this vehicle appears to be an ordinary mobile home. **B.** Inside it's a mobile drug lab. (*Courtesy Oregon State Fire Marshal's Office, Salem, OR*)

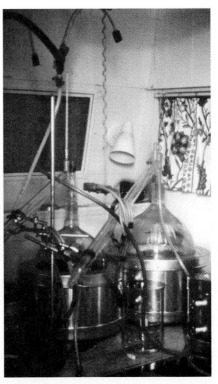

Figure 12-3 Clandestine drug lab with extensive glassware and sophisticated equipment. (*Courtesy Oregon State Fire Marshal's Office, Salem, OR*)

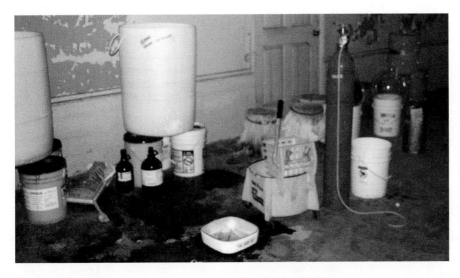

Figure 12-2 A lab capable of producing large quantities of methamphetamine.

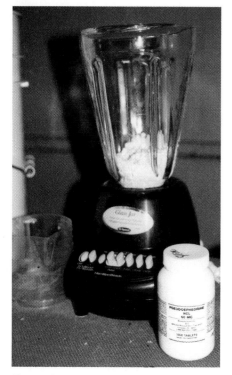

Figure 12-4 Ephedrine and pseudoephedrine tablets, available at any pharmacy, are ground in household blender as the first step in "meth" production.

and filtered through a coffee filter into a food canning jar (**Figure 12-4**). Reaction time is only 10 minutes. Other products that are used include anhydrous ammonia and either sodium or lithium metal, which is often extracted from camera batteries. This method also requires the use of solvents such as acetone and ether. This type of lab is also identified by the unusual quantities of "Coleman" fuel in the lab area. All of the necessary ingredients can be purchased at any discount department store and recipes are available over the Internet (**Table 12-1**).

An even simpler process is known as the "cold method," which does not require heat for the chemical reaction to occur. This method produces small quantities of product, approximately 1 ounce at a time. The process combines ephedrine or pseudoephedrine with two other chemicals, and takes approximately 3 hours to complete. The reaction vessel is made from two 32-ounce sports bottles (**Figure 12-5**).

Table 12-1 Materials Common to Methamphetamine Labs

Product	Chemical	Hazard
Aluminum foil	Aluminum	Nonhazardous
Camera batteries	Lithium	Water reactive
Charcoal lighter fluid	Petroleum	Flammable
Denaturer alcohol	Alcohol	Flammable
Epsom salts	Magnesium sulfate	Nonhazardous
Gasoline	Petroleum	Flammable
Heet	Methyl alcohol	Flammable
Iodine crystals	Iodine	Irritant
7% Tincture of Iodine	Iodine	Irritant
Kerosene	Petroleum	Flammable
Lacquer thinner	Petroleum	Flammable
Mineral spirits	Petroleum	Flammable
Muriatic acid	Hydrochloric acid	Corrosive acid
Red Devil Lye	Sulfuric acid	Corrosive base
Roto Rooter	Sulfuric acid	Corrosive acid
Starting Fluid	Ethyl ether	Flammable
Striker plates (fuses)	Phosphorus	Flammable
Table salt	Sodium chloride	Nonhazardous
Cold medications (over the counter)	Ephedrine and pseudoephedrine	Nonhazardous

Product	Use
Coffee filter, cheesecloth, napkins	Separate liquid from solids
Pots, pans, pressure cooker	Cooking
Iced tea jars, sports jars	Separating layers of liquids

Drug Enforcement Administration, Clandestine Laboratory Awareness, Pamphlet, Office of Training.

Fire and EMS personnel may be exposed to the dangers of an illegal drug lab if unsuspecting neighbors request the fire department to investigate unusual odors near their home. The odors produced during the drug production process in a P-2-P lab can be mistaken for the smell of dried cat urine, cat litter, or rotten garbage. Many chemicals are used during the mixing process, including ether, which has a distinctive smell that many people recognize and report when calling for assistance (**Figure 12-6**).

Because of the highly flammable properties of many of the chemicals stored in an illegal drug lab, the response to a building or vehicle fire may turn into an anything-but-normal situation. After a dwelling fire that had been especially difficult to extinguish, firefighters in northern California discovered over 200 5-gallon drums of chemicals. Nine of the firefighters were taken to the hospital after inhaling toxic fumes from the chemicals. The firefighters realized that the house was being used as a clandestine drug lab and requested law enforcement assistance. Further investigation produced a large amount of money, firearms and ammunition, and a cache of illegal drugs with a street value of $600,000.[6]

Because many illegal drug makers are also users, you may discover an illegal drug lab whenever you respond to a reported overdose. Buildings that contain an illegal drug lab often have windows covered with black plastic, cardboard, or paint (**Figure 12-7**). When you enter a building or vehicle to treat an overdose victim, look for glassware and other fundamental items that you might find in a high-school chemistry laboratory.

People who work in illegal drug labs may request medical assistance if they develop symptoms of exposure to toxic, corrosive, explosive, or flammable materials. A list of chemicals that you may encounter is included in Table 12-1.

Hazards Associated with Clandestine Drug Labs

Every lab has a different configuration. Although there are no books of plans for constructing the perfect lab at the local bookstore, with the advent of the Internet, many plans are just a few keystrokes away. Recipes for drugs are usually handed down from one operator to another, or found on web sites.

Everything associated with a clandestine drug lab is hazardous! Be careful where you walk and avoid touching anything except the patient. An action as simple as shutting off the tap-water supply to a cooling condenser can cause an explosion. Turning off the heat during a heat-induced chemical reaction is even more hazardous. Many chemical reactions must be shut down in stages, and only the operator may understand the shut-down process. The operator may not even be present. Because some cooking processes take as long as 72 hours to complete, and are hazardous as well, some operators will mix the ingredients and leave the area as soon as cooking begins.

To protect the operation, operators set booby traps. Outside mechanisms include fragmentation and incendiary devices (hand grenades and claymore mines) (**Figure 12-8**), animal traps, and impaling stakes. Inside traps include vicious dogs, poisonous snakes, fishhooks hung at eye

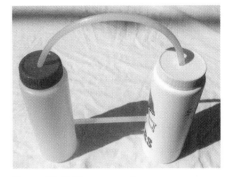

Figure 12-5 The unsuspecting emergency responder may not recognize this method of methamphetamine production.

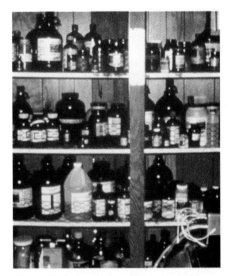

Figure 12-6 Chemical containers may not be properly labeled. *(Courtesy Oregon State Fire Marshal's Office, Salem, OR)*

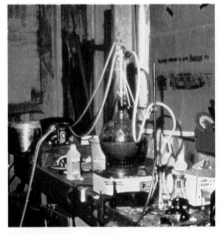

Figure 12-7 The cooker may cover windows with black plastic or cardboard to conceal his lab. *(Courtesy Oregon State Fire Marshal's Office, Salem, OR)*

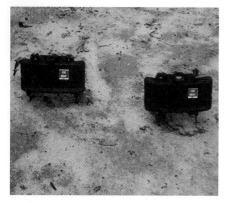

Figure 12-8 Claymore mines have been used as perimeter defense around the outside of labs.

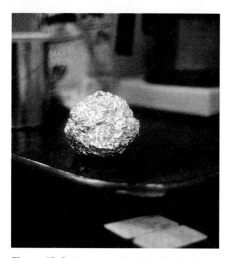

Figure 12-9 Upon exploding, this chemical booby trap can destroy a person's hand.

level, explosives connected to heating elements and electrical switches, and weapons such as crossbows and spear guns that discharge when the trigger mechanism is disturbed. Investigators have even found videotape cassettes containing plastic explosives and designed to detonate when placed in a video player.

Contact explosives are another danger you may face in an illegal drug lab.[7] These devices are made by combining potassium chlorate or red phosphorous with another chemical that becomes unstable when it dries. The chemicals are rolled into a ball of aluminum foil and placed throughout the laboratory. If the ball is disturbed, it will explode (**Figure 12-9**).

If possible, do not touch or move anything that you did not bring with you into the area. Never disturb a suspected booby trap! Mark the location and notify the incident commander of the device. Do not use a portable radio to notify the incident commander; a radio transmission may activate an explosive device. Go to the command post and tell the commander in person.

Emergency Scene Operations

All personnel and equipment used at the scene of an illegal drug lab will be contaminated. After the area has been identified as a clandestine lab, establish a preliminary hazardous materials hot zone. Include the lab and the surrounding area as well as all personnel and equipment that came in contact with the lab (**Figure 12-10**). If equipment has been removed from the lab and placed on a vehicle, include the vehicle in the hot zone. When the hazardous materials response team arrives on the scene, it will determine the final boundaries of the hot zone.

After you are clear of the building or vehicle containing the lab, notify your dispatcher that you are at the scene of an illegal drug lab,

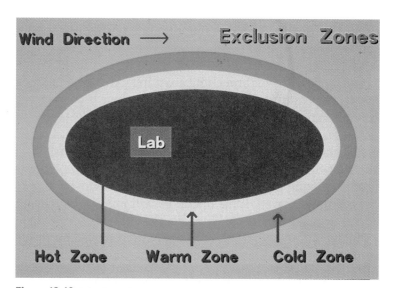

Figure 12-10 Establish safety zones for a hazardous materials response.

and request that the following agencies be notified to respond to the scene:

- Local law enforcement
- Drug Enforcement Administration
- Environmental Protection Agency
- Hazardous materials response team
- Additional EMS unit (ALS preferred)
- Bomb squad
- Local health department
- EMS supervisor
- Fire department for a full first-alarm response

EMS Operations

If you discover an illegal drug lab during an emergency medical call, leave the lab immediately. Take the patient with you if you can do so without exposing yourself and your team to additional hazardous materials. If the patient is stable, remain in the preliminary hot zone until the hazardous materials response team arrives on the scene. If your unit is outside the hot zone, do not return to it unless you need specific equipment for patient treatment. You, your partner, your patient, and all equipment carried into the lab are considered contaminated until cleared by the hazardous materials response team. Everyone and everything must be decontaminated before leaving the hot zone.

In an incident in Washington state, two people were operating a meth lab in an apartment. An explosion caused chemical burns to one of the operators. First responders, including two police officers and three emergency medical personnel, received treatment for eye irritation and respiratory distress. In addition, three hospital personnel were also incapacitated from exposure.[8]

The hazardous materials response team will set up and carry out decontamination procedures on *all* personnel and equipment leaving the hot zone. The decontamination stations are in a warm zone, which is adjacent to the hot zone. Access to the warm zone is limited to personnel directly involved in the incident.

If the patient's condition requires immediate transport to a hospital, notify the medical facility of the circumstances. Explain that you have been exposed to unknown hazardous materials and that you and the patient have not been decontaminated. Request that the hazardous materials response team be sent to the hospital to carry out decontamination procedures there. All hospital personnel and equipment that come into contact with you, the patient, or your equipment must be included in the decontamination procedure (**Figure 12-11**).

Fire Suppression Operations

If you respond to a fire that is in or around a suspected drug lab, you must wear full protective clothing, including positive-pressure breathing apparatus. Use higher levels of protective clothing, such as encapsulated suits, if chemicals are involved in the fire.

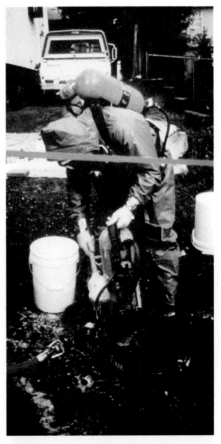

Figure 12-11 Proper protective clothing and complete decontamination must be part of standard operating procedures for clandestine drug lab operations. *(Courtesy Oregon State Fire Marshal's Office, Salem, OR)*

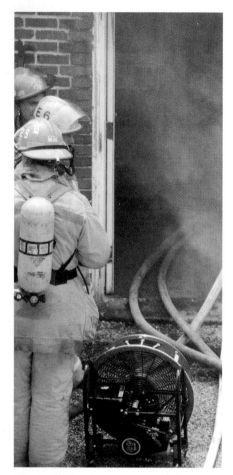

Figure 12-12 Positive-pressure ventilation is the only acceptable method of mechanical ventilation to use in drug lab operations. *(Courtesy Craig C. Schleunes)*

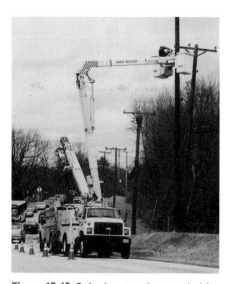

Figure 12-13 Trained personnel secure electric power to the suspected drug lab from a remote location.

Establish a hot zone as soon as possible. Again, access to the hot zone is limited to personnel directly involved in fire suppression. Personnel from other agencies that will handle the chemicals, protect the environment, and collect evidence are not allowed past the warm zone until after the fire is out or the fire ground commander specifically authorizes their presence.

Identify the warm zone as soon as the decontamination stations are erected. Backup personnel should move charged hose lines into the warm zone in anticipation of a rapid escalation of the fire. Backup should be properly positioned, fully bunkered, and ready to advance into the hot zone.

The area within the boundary of the fire line or crime scene tape and outside of the warm zone should be established as a *cold zone*. This controlled area is off-limits to the general public. The incident command post is located in this area. Protective clothing is not required, and the area may be used as a staging ground for additional personnel and equipment.

If the structure or vehicle containing a known lab is burning when you arrive, protect the exposures and *let it burn*. Attempting to control the fire may prove deadly to the fire attack teams. Remember, the runoff of contaminated water produced by suppression efforts may cause widespread ecological damage.

If an initial fire attack is in progress when the location is identified as a drug lab, withdraw the attack teams and shift from offensive to defensive operations.

In all incidents involving drug labs, evacuate the structures on every side of the incident. When a fire or chemical spill is involved, consider evacuating people downwind from the incident.

Positive-Pressure Ventilation

Never enter a known drug lab until the hazardous materials response team ventilates the area and declares it safe. All personnel responding to emergency medical situations, fire operations, chemical spills, and law enforcement activities should remain outside and upwind from the location.

Many of the chemicals used in clandestine drug labs are explosive if the proper air-to-product ratio is attained. Because this ratio will occur at some point during the ventilation process, all possible ignition sources must be eliminated.

If mechanical ventilation of the structure or vehicle is required, positive-pressure ventilation should be used. All mechanical and power equipment remain outside of the area being ventilated, which further reduces the number of ignition sources during the ventilation process (**Figure 12-12**).

Check with the DEA's on-scene chemist or site safety officer before turning off any utilities. Do not continue the operation until the DEA chemist arrives on the scene. After you receive permission from the chemist, secure all electric power from remote locations to prevent unwanted sparks or arcing (**Figure 12-13**).

To extinguish pilot lights on stoves, heaters, and furnaces, shut off all natural and low-pressure gas valves from outside the building. Do not shut off the gas if the DEA chemist believes that it is not safe to remove the heat from a chemical reaction in progress. It may be necessary to withdraw all personnel to the cold zone and wait until the process is complete.

Monitoring Personnel Working in the Hot Zone

An ALS unit (BLS unit if ALS is not available) should be assigned to all clandestine drug lab operations to monitor everyone working in the hot zone. The unit establishes a monitoring station in the warm zone. All personnel leaving the hot zone report to the monitoring station for medical evaluation after decontamination.

Provide medical attention to anyone who develops any of the following symptoms associated with exposure to toxic chemicals:

- Nausea
- Vomiting
- Sharp headache
- Reddened face
- Burning sensation in the nose, throat, or lungs
- Drowsiness
- Numb lips
- Tingling teeth
- Unfocused eyes (Sacramento Fire Department, Sacramento, CA, Clandestine Drug Lab Incidents: Procedures for HMRT, unpublished material, 1987)

Chemicals used in labs can be absorbed into the walls and floors of the building. This can create a potential health hazard that lasts days or weeks after a lab was dismantled and all chemicals and equipment removed from the site. The DEA posts warning signs on clandestine drug laboratories that have been seized and dismantled **(Figure 12-14)**.

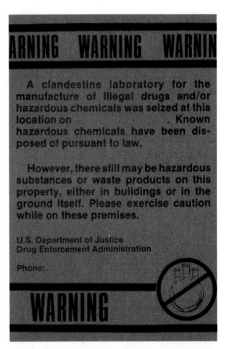

Figure 12-14 Whenever you see this sign, treat the area as if the laboratory were still operating.

Interacting with a Methamphetamine User

Methamphetamine is a powerful central nervous system stimulant that can be injected, snorted, smoked, or swallowed. Because the drug produces a sense of euphoria, increased alertness, and energy, it is popular with students, truck drivers and other professions that require long hours of work. Higher doses and chronic use of the drug will produce irritability and paranoia. If a patient is suspected of using meth, emergency responders should use the "interview stance" described in Chapter 13. However, you should remain 7' to 10' away from the individual and keep your hands visible at all times. If you move closer, the paranoid user may feel threatened and attempt an attack. You should also avoid shining lights into the eyes of a suspected meth user because this may also result in a violent attack. Speak slowly in a low-pitched voice. Any movement you make should also be slow and deliberate.[9]

Club Drugs

In recent years, a new drug problem has emerged throughout the country—club drugs. Although they are often seen in nightclub settings, club drugs are most prevalent at raves. Raves are after-hour

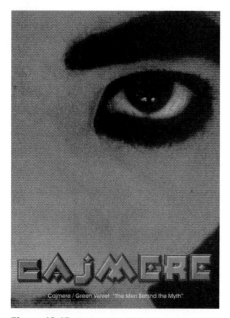

Figure 12-15 Poster advertising a rave.

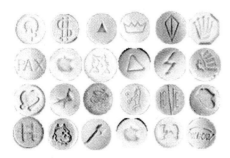

Figure 12-16 Logos on ecstasy pills.

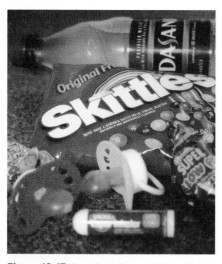

Figure 12-17 Paraphernalia associated with ecstasy use and raves.

parties where electronic or techno music is played, most often by DJs. A rave can last all night or one to two days (**Figure 12-15**). Some raves have been attended by more than 10,000 people. Drugs used at raves include Ecstasy, ketamine, GHB, and Rohypnol. Each can be easily acquired on the street, in schools, on college campuses, and over the Internet.

Ecstasy. Ecstasy (3,4-methylenedioxymethamphetamine, or MDMA) is rapidly gaining popularity with high school and college students from suburban enclaves to rural America. Many professionals are also using this drug in the nightclub setting believing that it is harmless. MDMA is also known as X, E, Adam, or XTC.

The bulk of MDMA is clandestinely produced in the Netherlands and Belgium for as little as $.50 per pill. It is then shipped to the United States, oftentimes through the mail or other parcel services, for distribution through illegal drug markets. The street price is $20 to $30 per pill.[10] Some clandestine labs producing Ecstasy have been found in the United States. Ecstasy pills are often marked with a brand name logo or symbol, such as a peace fish, a lightning bolt, a four-leaf clover, a bunny or a cartoon character (**Figure 12-16**). Ecstasy is often used in combination with other drugs, such as LSD, PCP, marijuana, methamphetamine, cocaine, and even Viagra.

In some aspects, MDMA is similar to amphetamine and methamphetamine. Because it produces a state of euphoria, extreme relaxation, and empathy for others, it has become known as the "hug drug" or the "feel-good" drug. Its effects last for 4 to 6 hours. Taking additional doses or "piggy-backing" can enable users to endure 2- to 3-day-long parties because the drug suppresses the need to sleep, eat, or drink. This can lead to severe dehydration, heat stroke, and possibly heart failure. Body-core temperatures can reach 107°F to 109°F, resulting in loss of consciousness and seizures.[11] Medical problems with this drug have forced some nightclubs to hire off-duty paramedics.[12]

Symptoms of an overdose include a rapid heart rate, high blood pressure, faintness, muscle cramping, seizures, panic attacks, and loss of consciousness. Muscle tension in the jaw and teeth grinding are side effects of MDMA, so many users often have lollypops or pacifiers in their mouths (**Figure 12-17**). To reduce muscle cramping, users will massage each other. Due to increased tactile sensitivity users can also be found spreading Vick's VapoRub over their body and using Vick's Inhalers.

LSD. One drug experiencing a resurgence in popularity is lysergic acid diethylamide, commonly referred to as LSD or acid. LSD is a powerful hallucinogenic drug that is popular at raves. Cookers of this drug will usually have far more chemistry background than the typical meth cooker because its production is more complex. The most popular method of distributing this drug is on blotter paper, thin sheets of paper dampened with the LSD and perforated into individual dosage units. A single dose sells for $4 to $5, although some are sold for as little as $1. Other popular methods of distribution include treated sugar cubes and small treated gelatin squares known as "window panes." It may also be distributed in small breath mint vials.

Large doses of LSD were initially popular in the 1960s. Today the dosage has been cut to help prevent unwanted reactions, but this has also contributed to its increasing popularity among young people. Flashbacks, or recurrences of the drug's effects, can still occur, even at the lower potency levels. Other side effects include panic, confusion, suspicion, and anxiety.[13]

Date-Rape Drugs. Law enforcement is seeing another disturbing trend in the nightclub scene: the use of "date-rape" drugs. Rohypnol, ketamine, and gamma-hydroxybutyrate are being used to incapacitate unsuspecting male and female victims. The amnesia produced by each of these drugs makes prosecution of the suspected rapist difficult because most victims cannot recall the circumstances of the incident.

Ketamine, also known as "K" or "Special K," is an anesthetic used in both humans and animals. Many veterinary clinics are being robbed for their stock of ketamine. In small doses it is a club drug with effects similar to PCP and LSD that last an hour or less. Higher doses can lead to a "near-death" or "out-of-body" experience. It can also cause fatal respiratory complications.[14]

Gamma-hydroxybutyrate (GHB), a central nervous system depressant, is sometimes known on the street as "liquid x," "easy lay," "gamma-oh," and "soap." This drug remains popular with some body builders because it allegedly stimulates muscle growth. In small doses, GHB causes dizziness, drowsiness, nausea, and visual disturbances. Larger doses can result in seizures, acute respiratory depression, unconsciousness, and coma. It is easily made by mixing caustic soda with gamma-butyrolactone (GBL), a chemical found in some paint strippers. This produces a colorless, odorless liquid with a slightly salty taste, that is difficult to detect when placed in a person's drink. Adding GBH to alcohol increases the probability of respiratory difficulty. As of January 2000, 60 deaths have been attributed to GHB.[15] In early February 1999, the small town of Salisbury, Maryland, had five GHB overdoses in one week. One victim nearly died.[16] GHB is often carried in small bottles of mouthwash or eyedrops.

The third type of date-rape drug is flunitrazepam, which is marketed under the trade name Rohypnol. It is legal and widely available in Europe and Latin America to treat insomnia; it is typically smuggled into the United States through the mail and other parcel services. Street names include "roofies" and "forget-me-pill." It is more powerful than Valium and can cause decreased blood pressure, drowsiness, confusion, dizziness, visual disturbances, decreased respirations, coma, and gastrointestinal difficulties. In sexual assault cases the drug cannot be detected by normal screening procedures.

These new lines of illegal substances, along with the continued popularity of marijuana, heroin, and crack cocaine, will result in an increase in substance abuse cases being seen by prehospital providers. Due to the seriousness of the problem at raves, law enforcement suggests that multiple ALS units be staged at these events. Information on planning for these events can be found in Chapter 14.

SURVIVAL TIPS

1 Clandestine drug labs are extremely dangerous. Do not enter known labs until they have been secured by law enforcement personnel. All personnel and agencies responding to an incident at an illegal drug lab need an immediate plan of action. Liquid propane gas cylinders routinely used with home barbecues are now being used to hold anhydrous ammonia, a necessary chemical in the production of methamphetamine. Responders should be aware that anhydrous ammonia will react with the brass fittings of the cylinder. The reaction will cause a blue tinge on the valve and will result in failure of the container.

2 The time to plan for multiagency operations is not when a clandestine drug lab is discovered—it is now!

3 A drug lab is a crime scene—preserve the evidence!

4 Limit overhaul to extinguishing serious hot spots that may reignite or ignite residue vapors.

5 When use of a date-rape drug is suspected in a sexual assault case, ask the victim to delay urinating until a sample can be taken and analyzed. Traces of the drug may be identifiable in urine. For other standard evidence preservation techniques, see Chapter 16.

Chapter 13

Self-Defense Tactics

Recognizing the potential for violence when you arrive on the scene gives you the opportunity to get support and protection. With assistance from law enforcement, you should be able to treat your patient safely after the scene is secure. However, you must also consider what to do if the violence is ongoing or breaks out while you are delivering care. If you know some effective defensive moves, you may be able to resolve the situation without getting hurt yourself.

What should you do if the patient is being assaulted when you arrive? Should you jump in the middle of the fracas and protect the patient from harm? How would you react if an attack occurred while you or your crew were providing patient care?

One response to these questions is "Assist the assailant with oxygen therapy." This does not mean using a nasal cannula; instead, it refers to hitting the assailant on the head with a "D" cylinder. Although this technique is very effective, it opens the door for lawsuits against the responder and the agency.

There are other alternatives. You may be able to use your voice to bring the incident under control (see Chapter 7). But if the aggressor ignores your voice commands and continues to press forward, what action should you take? Should you use force against someone who is trying to hurt you or prevent you from reaching a patient?

Reasonable Use of Force

A reasonable level of force is the minimum amount of force needed to accomplish a goal. Emergency service providers can use a reasonable level of force to accomplish the following goals:

- Reach and treat any patient who is not breathing or who has a blocked airway.

- Reach and treat any patient who is in cardiac arrest and could die without immediate corrective action.
- Reach and treat any patient with severe trauma.
- Remove any person who interferes with life-saving patient care.
- Move any person who attempts to prevent your retreat from a dangerous situation.

When you are faced with a situation that requires the use of force, always start with a verbal challenge. Do not grab a person by the arm and pull. Physical contact with people is no longer acceptable conduct for emergency service workers as an initial line of defense.

If someone prevents you from reaching your patient, identify yourself and say, "Move back! That person may die if you don't let me help!" If the person blocking your way moves, you have attained your goal and no additional force is required. If the person does not move, take a side step and repeat the verbal challenge. Inform the person, "If you don't get out of my way, I'm calling the police!" This threat usually makes the person move, but not always in the direction you wished. Be prepared to defend yourself.

Use physical force as a defensive technique, not an aggressive motion. Properly executed defensive motions can be as effective as physical strikes and are easier to defend if you face civil liability charges.

The amount of defensive force needed to protect yourself varies with each incident. If you feel that your life is in imminent danger,

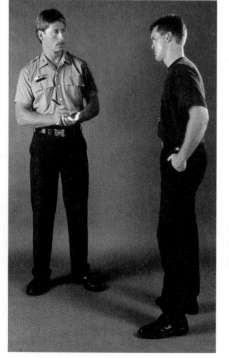

Figure 13-1 The interview stance.

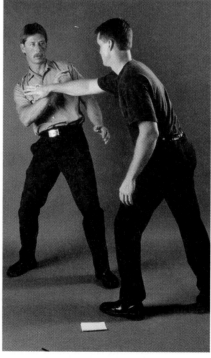

Figure 13-2 The interview stance facilitates balance and rapid movement to a more defensible position.

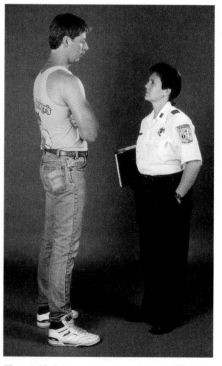

Figure 13-3 Do not stand with your feet together or with your hands in your pockets when talking to a stranger.

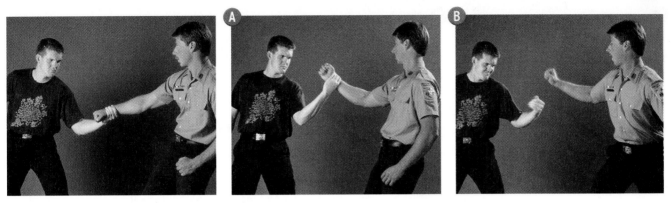

Figure 13-4 The normal reaction is to pull away.   **Figure 13-5 A.** Pull toward the thumb. **B.** Break the hold, turn, and run.

any action that gets you out of the situation is a reasonable level of force.

The Interview Stance

If you are prepared, you can control an unexpected attack. Always use the interview stance so you will be in a defensive position if violence suddenly erupts. This stance is especially helpful in domestic encounters (see Chapter 9).

To assume the interview stance, stand approximately an arm's length from the person with your body at a 45° angle to the person. Your feet should be shoulder-width apart, your knees slightly bent, and your hands relaxed (**Figure 13-1**).

Look relaxed when you talk to the person. An unnatural stance signals that you are prepared for trouble and may cause the person to become aggressive (**Figure 13-2**).

If you practice, this stance will be automatic when you talk with a civilian. It is a comfortable way to stand and much safer than standing with your feet close together and facing the other person (**Figure 13-3**).

The Wrist Grasp

If someone unexpectedly grabs your wrists, your normal reaction is to pull away or jerk back from the attacker. However, you should be aware of both the grip and the direction in which you move. If you try to break the grip by pulling against the assailant's fingers, you will have difficulty in breaking the hold (**Figure 13-4**). But if you jerk your forearm against the assailant's thumb (**Figure 13-5**), you can easily break free. Usually this means you will pull toward your body instead of away from it. This move is more effective because the thumb is weaker than the combined strength of the fingers (**Figure 13-6**). Once you are free of the assailant's grip, retreat to a safe area.

Technique for Distracting an Assailant

If an assailant grabs the front of your shirt, seize the hand of the attacker and twist it toward the thumb. At the same time, flash your free hand through the assailant's field of vision. This unexpected action

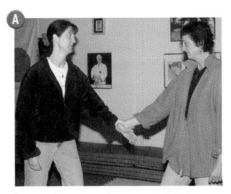

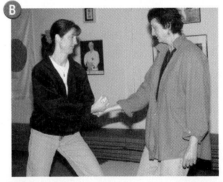

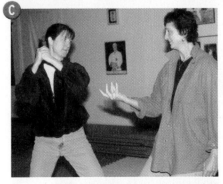

Figure 13-6 A. The attacker's grip is too strong for you to pull free when pulling against the fingers. **B.** Use your free hand to increase your pulling power. **C.** Reach between you and your assailant, grab your trapped hand, and pull yourself free.

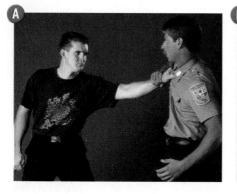
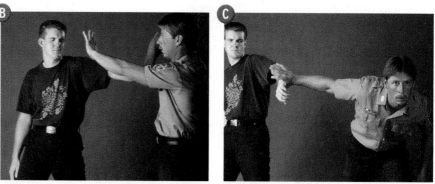

Figure 13-7 **A.** Seize your attacker's hand and twist toward the thumb. **B.** Flash your free hand in your attacker's face, which will break the concentration long enough for you to escape. **C.** After you feel the grip relaxing on your shirt, twist your body away from your assailant and run to a safer area.

should break the person's concentration long enough for you to break the hold and escape (**Figure 13-7**).

The Power of a Tweak

A tweak is performed by pinching a small piece of skin under a person's upper arm. If you pinch, twist, and pull at the same time, you can bring most people to their knees, regardless of size. This move is most painful when applied directly to the skin (**Figure 13-8**). If the assailant is wearing a long-sleeved shirt or jacket, a tweak may not be effective.

Breaking a Headlock

What if your assailant grabs you and holds you in a headlock? Your most effective move is to reach up to the attacker's head and place you first two fingers just above the lip and under the nose. Now apply pressure under the nose, lifting the upper lip up and back. This is not only painful, it will also forcing the assailant's head backward (**Figure 13-9**). Your attacker will release the hold and you will be able to escape.

Breaking a Stranglehold When Attacked from the Front

If an assailant tries to strangle you from the front, raise both arms outward from the sides of your body. Rotate either arm in a windmill motion, using your upper arm to hit the assailant's wrist and break the hold. Do this movement quickly and with as much physical force as possible (**Figure 13-10**).

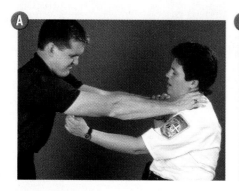
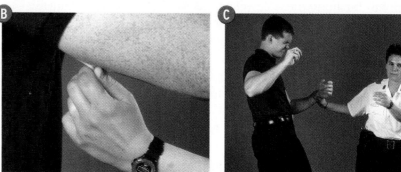

Figure 13-8 **A.** One way to break a front stranglehold is to apply a tweak. **B.** Pinch, pull, and twist a small piece of skin under the arm. **C.** As soon as you feel the assailant's grip relax, twist and run.

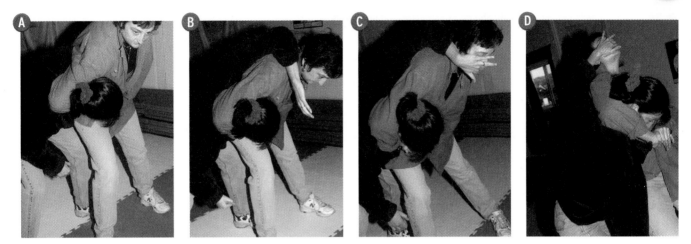

Figure 13-9 A. An attacker puts you in a headlock. **B.** Your right arm should come up toward the assailant's head. **C.** Use the index and middle fingers to put pressure on the area below the nose and above the lip. **D.** Continue applying pressure upward and backward. The attacker will loosen the head-lock as her neck hyperextends.

Breaking a Stranglehold Applied from the Rear

If your assailant places a right arm around your neck, use both of your hands to pull the assailant's forearm toward your chest. At the same time, drop to your right knee and twist your body to the left. Your assailant will lose balance and be thrown to the ground directly in front of you. As soon as the hold is broken, get up and run (**Figure 13-11**).

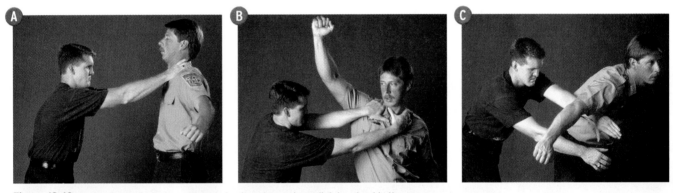

Figure 13-10 A. If someone facing you attempts to strangle you, immediately extend both arms. **B.** Rotate either arm in a windmill motion to break the hold. **C.** As soon as you break the hold, run.

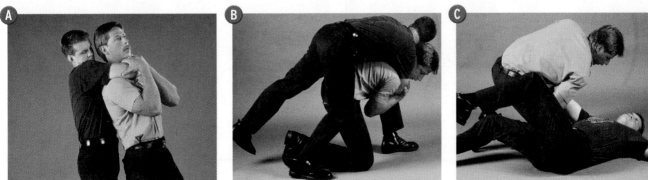
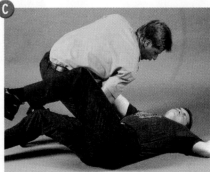

Figure 13-11 A. If you are attacked from the right, grab your assailant's right forearm and pull toward your chest. **B.** At the same time, drop to your right knee and turn your body toward the assailant. **C.** Once you break the hold, get up and run.

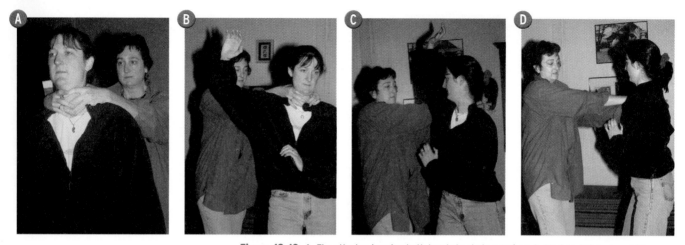

Figure 13-12 A. The attacker is using both hands to choke you from behind. **B.** Raise your right arm. **C.** As the arm continues upward, rotate your upper body backward. **D.** Continue to spin backward, which will cause the assailant to lose his grip.

If your assailant places a left arm around your neck, drop to your left knee while pulling the assailant's left forearm toward your chest and twisting your body to the right. The result will be the same. The assailant will be thrown off-balance and land on the ground in front of you.

Defending Against a Choke Hold from Behind

If your assailant grabs your neck from behind and attempts to choke you, raise your arm and rotate your upper body to face the assailant (**Figure 13-12**). The assailant will be unable to maintain the choke hold. You need to make this move very quickly because a choke hold can cut off the supply of oxygen to the lungs and the supply of oxygenated blood to the brain, resulting in unconsciousness.

Breaking a Rear Bear Hug

If you are engulfed by a bear hug, with your attacker behind you, you can free yourself even if your arms are pinned to your side.

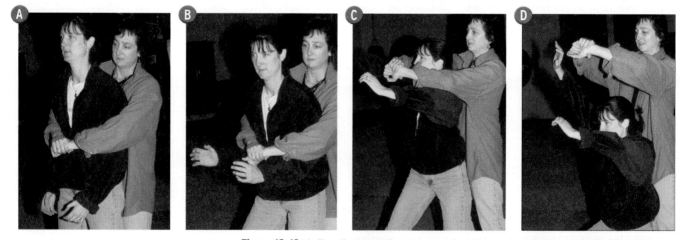

Figure 13-13 A. The attacker applies a bear hug from the rear trapping your arms. **B.** Raise your arms upward. **C.** Continue the upward motion as you begin to drop toward the floor. **D.** When you reach a squatting position, lunge forward to escape the hold.

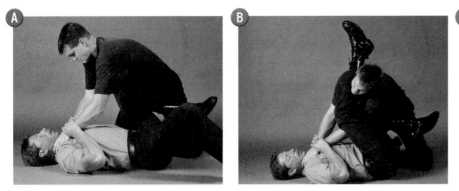

Figure 13-14 A. To break a stranglehold from above, bring your right knee up against the assailant's hip or stomach and grab both of the assailant's wrists. **B.** Swing your left leg up, hook it under the assailant's chin, and push toward the ground. **C.** This loosens your assailant's grip on your throat and pushes him backward to the ground so you can escape to a safer area.

Maintain your balance as you raise your arms. Continue to thrust your arms upward and quickly stoop toward the floor (**Figure 13-13**). As you drop toward the floor, begin to move in a forward direction so you can make a quick escape once you are free.

Breaking a Stranglehold Applied from Above

You may often find that your patient is on the floor or ground. In some cases, you may even move the patient to the ground or floor. However, this means that to provide patient care, you must kneel or squat next to the patient. In either position, you are very vulnerable to an unexpected attack from above. An assailant can easily gain a stranglehold and wrestle you to the ground.

In **Figure 13-14**, an assailant is strangling a paramedic after attacking him from the right. The paramedic uses the leg-bar technique to break free. To break a stranglehold from above, bring your right knee up against the assailant's hip or stomach and grab both of the assailant's wrists. Swing your left leg up, hook it under the assailant's chin, and push toward the ground. This loosens your assailant's grip on your throat and pushes him backward to the ground so you can escape to a safer area.

Defending Yourself When Knocked to the Ground

If you must defend yourself after being knocked to the ground, use your feet and legs to guard against strikes and blows to your lower body (**Figure 13-15 A-B**). Use your hands and arms to block strikes to the upper body (**Figure 13-15 C**). At the first opportunity, get to your feet and retreat to a safe area.

Practice

The self-defense tactics presented in this chapter can save your life if they are properly applied. The only way you will learn to apply these techniques correctly is to practice each one under controlled conditions. You must practice until you can do every motion without thinking. A qualified instructor should supervise practice sessions until you master the techniques. After you have mastered these techniques, continue to

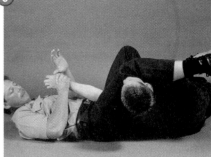

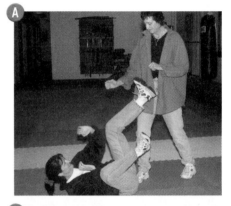

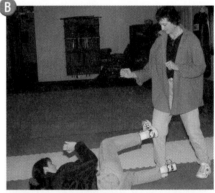

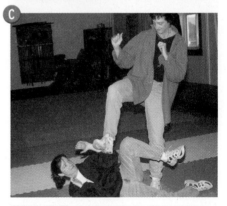

Figure 13-15 A. You are on the ground and an assailant is attempting to attack. **B.** Use your feet and legs to ward off attacks to the lower body. **C.** Use your arms and hands to defend against blows to the upper body.

practice so that you can maintain both your skill level and your automatic response. Your reaction to attack must be immediate and automatic. If violence erupts, you will not have time to think; you will have to act.

Documentation

Report any threatened or actual assaults to the police. Even if the incident seemed insignificant, file a police report.

If you had to defend yourself and used one of the techniques presented in this chapter, state the facts clearly and completely in the police report. Anytime you put your hands on someone during the course of your duties for reasons other than providing patient care, ensure that the reasons are documented, placed on file, and available for use in case of litigation.

SURVIVAL TIPS

1. You do not have the authority, training, or responsibility to subdue a person who is preventing you from reaching your patient. That is the police department's responsibility.

2. If you recognize that the patient will die without immediate treatment, use verbal force to gain access to the patient. If you fail to reach the patient, call for police assistance, be extremely forceful in your verbal demands, and be ready to defend yourself.

3. Know the local laws regarding the use of force by fire and EMS personnel.

4. Never carry or use an unauthorized weapon to defend yourself or your patient.

5. Remember, you can be sued for any action you take. Individual departments must formulate written policies to protect personnel who are involved in a physical confrontation during the course of their duties.

6. When you use the self-defense techniques presented in this chapter, use them with all the physical strength you possess. You are fighting for your life!

Chapter 14

Tactical Emergency Medical Support

The first edition of this text included a chapter on "SWAT Medics." Since then, however, the role of the SWAT medic has expanded into a specialty of its own. Today most firefighters and EMTs refer to it as Tactical Emergency Medical Support (TEMS).

Fire, rescue, and EMS personnel routinely find themselves in life-threatening situations. This may involve rescuing a young child from a burning house, controlling a chemical leak at a HazMat incident, or extricating the driver from a vehicle hanging precariously over a cliff. Fire and rescue services have become very proficient in handling such emergencies.

Fire and rescue personnel may also be needed at civil disturbances, areas where suspected criminals are barricaded, hostage situations, and other potentially explosive incidents. All of these situations are law enforcement problems and are usually handled by a law enforcement agency. The police operate inside a clearly identified police zone, and fire suppression and EMS personnel wait outside in a staging area unless needed.

If a situation suddenly deteriorates and someone is injured, or if the police need special assistance from fire suppression personnel, teams may be called from the controlled staging area and asked to enter a potentially dangerous police zone. But attempting an ad hoc rescue without special training in a situation already spinning out of control can be disastrous and deadly. Most fire, rescue, and EMS personnel thrust into this situation are not trained to operate under these conditions, against armed assailants. In addition, most firefighters and EMTs have no interest in receiving the training, and should not be expected to perform such duties. The National Fire Protection Association's "Standard on Fire Department Occupational Safety and Health Program" (NFPA 1500) states, "Fire department companies or teams that provide support to law enforcement agency special weapons and tactics (SWAT)

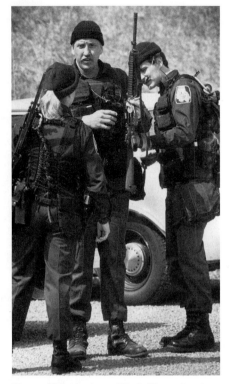

Figure 14-1 Members of the Baltimore County SWAT team check their gear before taking their positions during a hostage situation. (*Courtesy Charles Weiss, Patuxent Publishing Company, Columbia, MD*)

operations shall receive special training." Fire, rescue, and EMS personnel who have not received specialized SWAT training *must* remain outside of the SWAT team's operating perimeter (**Figure 14-1**).

Special Weapons and Tactics (SWAT) teams were established in 1966 by the Los Angeles Police Department and the Los Angeles County Sheriff's Department, following a summer of riots. Since then, many other jurisdictions developed SWAT teams. The small-unit tactics used by these teams were initially drawn from the military. Today, many tactics developed by SWAT teams from across the country are being used by the military.

The Team

Although combat-ready military units will not deploy without some type of medical support, until recently the same could not be said of many law enforcement tactical teams. The Los Angeles County Sheriff's Department began assigning medics to their SWAT teams in 1974. Hundreds of agencies now employ some type of medical system to support their specialized tactical units. No national standards for recognition as a tactical medic exist, and team size and configuration vary depending on local needs. In some cases, SWAT team operators are trained as emergency medical technicians; in other cases, a trained physician may serve as a team officer. Between these options are a variety of alternatives, each with its own advantages and disadvantages. Most teams, however, use some type of advanced life support provider as their tactical medic.

From experience, many teams will readily admit that having team members as medics simply does not work. In one instance, a team had trained a number of their personnel as emergency medical technicians. One of the emergency medical technicians was a countersniper; the other was the point man on the assault team. But in an actual situation, the countersniper could not be expected to relinquish his primary responsibility and provide medical care. Nor could the point man be expected to provide medical care, particularly because, as the first person through the door, he would be the most likely candidate to be injured. Team members cannot focus on their law enforcement mission and a medical mission at the same time. Thus, many departments have elected to employ fire/rescue emergency medical technicians to support the medical mission. By doing so, tactical officers can focus on the law enforcement mission and the emergency medical technicians can concentrate on medical issues surrounding the incident.

Regardless of the team/medic configuration, tactical medics must have an intimate knowledge of all SWAT team operating procedures. Medics must also understand the criminal's reaction to SWAT team activities so that they can determine the necessary procedures for effective patient care. In some incidents, a patient cannot be moved until the situation is stabilized. The tactical medic must be emotionally and professionally prepared to provide quality patient care in an unstable environment.

Tactical medics, as well as all SWAT team members, spend countless off-duty hours engaged in physical conditioning. In addition to the usual fire, rescue, EMS, or law enforcement duties, they must also develop and maintain the unique skills required for the diverse missions they face.

Goals of a TEMS Program

The goals of a TEMS program are multifaceted. Obviously, any such program would attempt to reduce death and injury to police officers as well as innocent bystanders and suspects (**Figure 14-2**). Other goals are not as obvious. Appropriately trained tactical medics will reduce a police department's injury and disability costs by providing quick, efficient medical care to SWAT officers whether they are on a mission or in training. A by-product is improved morale. Both tactical team members and regular patrol officers will feel that their agency command staff care about their welfare. Finally, a trained medical unit reduces the possibility of successful litigation against a police agency for inappropriate medical care to a suspect or victim in a barricade or hostage situation.

Medics are a valuable resource for the law enforcement incident commander. Their role involves far more than just on-scene medical care (**Figure 14-3**). Tactical medics are also responsible for the overall health and welfare of the entire team. They are invaluable in gathering intelligence about the medical condition of barricaded subjects, hostages, and hostage takers. Their interaction with hostage negotiators can be pivotal in the outcome of the situation. Specifically, they are responsible for:

- Acquiring and maintaining pertinent medical histories of team members. When a member is injured, the medic is responsible for transferring this information to the receiving medical facility.

- Observing and monitoring team members for adverse effects resulting from prolonged operations, hazardous conditions, and inclement weather.

- Providing the most appropriate emergency and nonemergency care to anyone who might become sick or injured during a tactical operation or training mission.

- Serving as liaisons between an injured team member's family, the law enforcement agency, and the medical facility. The medic is

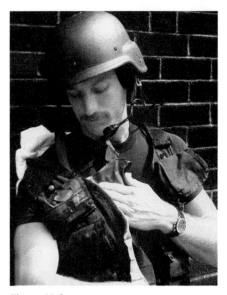

Figure 14-2 The goal of a Tactical Emergency Medical Support program is to reduce mortality and morbidity among police officers, innocent civilians, and suspects involved in tactical law enforcement missions.

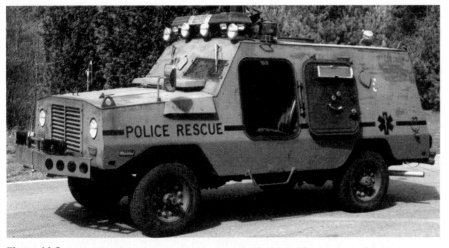

Figure 14-3 Armored personnel carrier used to evacuate the injured from unsecured areas.

responsible for keeping command officers and family informed about the officer's medical condition.

- Conducting medical mission planning for each operation.

Although a number of agencies arm their medics, the medics are not considered an aggressive part of an assault team. Their presence is for immediate medical care in a hostile environment. Weapons assigned to tactical medics are used only in self-defense. The arming of medics is a sensitive issue that should be carefully broached with the SWAT team leader. One way to handle this issue may be to teach tactical medics how to "safe" all weapons carried by the team. Then, if an officer is injured, the medic will be capable of securing his or her weapon. In addition, the medics can be taught how to use each of the weapons, in the event of an emergency that requires the medic to defend himself or herself.

Training

The intensity of emergency medical training and the amount of police training required for fire, rescue, and EMS personnel to qualify as tactical medics are determined by the authority having jurisdiction over the SWAT team. Several jurisdictions require medics to become certified as reserve officers or special deputies. Other jurisdictions require their tactical medics to attend a 120-hour SWAT school, but others have developed condensed courses to acclimate the medic to the tactical environment. Medics may receive extensive training in specific skills, depending on local conditions. For example, teams operating in metropolitan areas may focus on techniques of rappelling from helicopters and buildings, while teams in rural areas may spend more time on the techniques of land navigation.

There are a number of private concerns that provide specialized medical training for emergency medical technicians assigned to special operations teams. The premiere program, however, remains the Counter Narcotics Terrorism Operations Medical Support (CONTOMS) program. This 52-hour program is funded by the Department of Defense and covers a variety of topics including: mission planning, wound ballistics, preventative medicine, care under fire, and medicine across the barricade (**Figure 14-4**).

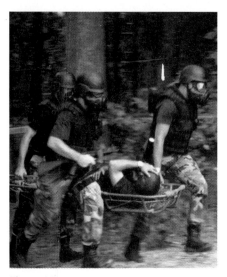

Figure 14-4 Tactical medics evacuate simulated patient during training mission.

Mission Planning

For years, fire services have conducted prefire planning or preincident surveys. During these surveys, the local engine company visits a target hazard to conduct a detailed assessment of the structure. Personnel gather information on air handling systems, building contents, elevators, exit locations, fire protection systems, and other factors from building occupants and design engineers. The fire department then attempts to anticipate the potential for fire spread and smoke travel. The company officer begins to formulate a plan of action if a call comes in from this address. In recent years, tactical medics have also been doing preincident planning prior to a known event such as a raid or executive protection detail. During this threat assessment or mission plan, they collect a variety of information and formulate a written plan.

In actuality, such planning is beneficial for any type of unusual or special event, whether it be a country music show or, in the case of a tactical medic, a raid or hostage rescue. Planning should begin as soon as your agency is notified of an event or mission. Many jurisdictions require permits for any large gathering. Make sure your agency is on the notification list when these permits are issued.

The information process begins with the obvious: date, time, and type of event. The plan is customized to the type of event. Is it an air show, a Neo-Nazi or similar demonstration, a triathlon, or a line-of-duty funeral for a police officer? How many people are expected to attend? A raid may target a single individual; there may be 1,000 to 2,000 people at the police officer's funeral, and up to 20,000 people may attend an air show. Events in Washington, DC, have attracted 250,000 to 500,000 attendees.

In some situations, a visit to the site may be needed, along with a site map. The amount of detail necessary will be dictated by the situation, and could range from a generalized plot plan for an outdoor event to one that resembles a prefire plan, with floor plans and exits, for an interior event. Tactical medics planning for a law enforcement mission will rely on the site maps developed by the police.

Each plan should have a designated landing zone (LZ) for any air evacuations that may be necessary. This may seem foolish when planning for some events, but it is always better to be prepared for the unexpected. In one incident, a planner included LZs in the plan for a police officer's funeral. Many police departments deploy SWAT teams as security during these funerals, and the planner realized that it would be an opportune time for someone to ambush a large number of officers at once! It is always better to prepare for the worst, and hope for the best.

If a Global Positioning System (GPS) unit is available, the latitude and longitude of each site in the plan should be noted. In some cases, more than one LZ may be needed. For example, the plan for a potentially violent demonstration at a state capitol had both a primary LZ and a secondary LZ. The primary LZ, closer to the site, was designated as "hot." This site would not be secured by law enforcement and might be compromised if violence erupted. The secondary LZ was designated as "cold." This site was on a secured military installation and would be used if the primary LZ was compromised.

This portion of the plan necessitates meeting with the agency or company providing the aeromedical service. In the state capitol example, it was also necessary to meet with the commanding officer, or his designee, of the military installation. Without advance warning, the military might have used antiaircraft fire when an unknown aircraft attempted to land at the installation. Landing an air ambulance helicopter in the middle of an airshow may also present a few challenges. Ground routes and travel time to each LZ should be part of the plan to avoid any conflicts with road closures, bridge outages, or other disruptions. This will also be helpful to any on-scene units from a distant response district that are not totally familiar with the area. If necessary, a map should be included in the final document.

The plan should also consider which medical facilities will be used. It should include a primary and secondary hospital, a trauma center, a burn center, and a pediatric center. Other specialty facilities can be added as necessary. Document the address of each facility, route of travel and travel time from the event site. A computer-based mapping program can be used to generate single-page maps in the final document, which will be helpful for units unfamiliar with the area.

Both the primary and secondary hospitals should be notified in advance of any special events that could have an impact on their admissions. Generally, the emergency department administrator is a good contact. The hospital should be aware of the specifics of the upcoming event, including any details on anticipated problems or hazards. If a rally or demonstration has the potential for violence, a representative from law enforcement should also be involved in meeting with hospital personnel.

In certain cases, law enforcement may wish to restrict the dissemination of sensitive information. Tactical medics must be especially careful to not divulge information about upcoming raids. The raid on the Branch Davidian compound in Waco, Texas, was compromised by a private ambulance company requested to standby at the site. Information on the raid was improperly released and discovered by the Davidians.

Reconsider the example of the demonstration at the state capitol. The closest hospital was only one block from the event site. The entry doors to the emergency department opened onto the main thoroughfare. If the situation exploded, the emergency department could have been overwhelmed with walk-in patients. A meeting between law enforcement officials and emergency department staff could identify some potential problems at the facility and provide suggestions to minimize or alleviate certain risks. With sufficient information, the hospital can conduct its own assessment and devise an appropriate plan. Hospital staff may also provide valuable input and resources for the tactical plan.

Continue to gather as much information as possible concerning the event. Has the event been held in previous years? Have police served high-risk warrants at the target address before? What is the history of the event? Have there been problems? Has the group planning the protest held demonstrations in other jurisdictions? A phone call to another fire department or EMS service familiar with handling demonstrations may prove fruitful. They can provide details on strategies and tactics that worked for them and warnings about pitfalls to avoid.

Identify as many hazards as possible, and do not overlook the weather. Extreme heat, humidity, or cold can have a major impact on the number of sick or injured from an event. Hundreds of young people succumbed to heat while on a pilgrimage with the Pope in Colorado a number of years ago. There are many web sites such as *www.weather.com* that provide short- and long-range forecasts. These sites also have both heat index and wind chill charts, which are helpful in predicting extreme conditions. Note the anticipated conditions in the written plan.

What other hazards can be anticipated? That may depend on the type of event. At an air show, there might be a plane crash; at a Ku Klux Klan rally, someone might inadvertently get pepper spray in the eyes.

One team of fire department divers standing by at a boat race were surprised when someone attempted suicide by jumping from the bridge above them.

Part of the planning process should also include identification of what resources will be necessary. The answer isn't always to add ALS units, engine companies, or staff officers. Depending on the circumstances, it may be more appropriate to have two transport units supplemented by medics on bicycles. Can a specially equipped golf cart be used? If it is necessary to have a fire department engine company on the scene, can a paramedic engine company be used? Are agencies other than traditionally based fire/EMS, such as the Red Cross, available to assist?

At a summer country music fair where the temperature is expected to be 100° with high humidity, strategically located water stations may be appropriate. Perhaps the on-scene engine company can set up a misting fan. This is also very useful for cooling marchers at the end of a parade. Using the public address system to make announcements on the need for continued hydration can significantly reduce the number of potential heat exhaustion cases.

The rally at the state capitol may require a decontamination station. Demonstrators who have been exposed to tear gas or pepper spray can be brought to the decontamination station before they are transported for any medical treatment. Tactical medics may be needed with separate secure areas for treating police officers and demonstrators. Treatment areas for law enforcement should be separate from those for detainees, and all police officers should be treated at one designated facility if possible. If the group throws vials of blood at the demonstrations, there should be on-scene measures available to quickly determine whether vials contain contaminated human blood, animal blood, or simply colored water.

Once all potential problems are identified, the material should be reviewed by someone else. Remember that if anything can go wrong, it probably will go wrong, and be prepared to respond. Although resources may not be available for every potential problem, identifying the problems will ensure that the document is as complete as possible. It will also help ensure that a call for additional resources will be quicker and more appropriate in size and structure.

Compile the material into a cohesive document. All associated agencies should have a copy of the plan. Do not forget to include responders from your own agency in the planning process. They may have unique solutions to complicated problems.

Fire and EMS units are routinely asked to serve at nontraditional venues, including tactical maneuvers. If all those involved have a copy of a written plan, the community will receive quick, appropriate service and the overall impact to sometimes beleaguered delivery systems will be reduced.

The role of the tactical medic is wide and varied. They support multiple missions such as providing executive protection, disposing of explosives, attending to barricade and hostage incidents, as well as delivering high-risk warrant service. The medical skills employed by these highly

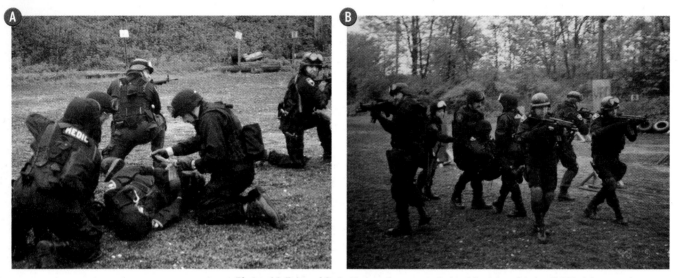

Figure 14-5 A and B Tactical medics prepare to treat the injured during field training exercise. *(Courtesy Union County Emergency Response Team)*

trained personnel are also controversial. Due to the violent circumstances, typical emergency medical care can actually endanger the emergency medical technician. Medical care more akin to battlefield medicine is practiced to ensure the lives of the tactical medics. Yet, data show that tactical medics have an impact by reducing death and injury to law enforcement officers and innocent civilians (**Figure 14-5**). Most importantly, using specially trained individuals reduces the possibility that untrained and unprepared emergency responders will be caught in the crossfire.

SURVIVAL TIPS

1 The National Fire Protection Association Standard 1500, *Fire Department Occupational and Health Program* states, "Fire department companies or teams that provide support to law enforcement agency special weapons and tactics (SWAT) operations shall receive special training." If you do not have such specialized training, do not enter the operating perimeter of such an incident.

2 Civil disturbances, mass-casualty shootings, acts of terrorism, and barricade and hostage incidents have changed the role of EMS. Agencies must adapt to the changes in society so that the EMS delivery system is capable of functioning appropriately during a crisis.

Chapter 15

Mass-Casualty Shootings

Mass-casualty shootings at businesses and schools are becoming common news stories. Even fire stations have experienced such violence. On April 24, 1996, a Jackson, Mississippi, firefighter went on a shooting rampage in the central fire station and killed four fire department officers. See **Box 15-1** on Mass-Casualty Shootings for a list of some of the mass shooting incidents that have occurred in recent years.

During the mass shooting incident at Columbine High School in Littleton, Colorado, police officers crouched behind a fire department engine company. They used the unit as protection when approaching the building. Fire and EMS are an integral part of emergency operations at these scenes. Yet, even though such incidents are becoming more frequent, many fire and EMS agencies have failed to develop response plans for these disasters. It is unrealistic and neglectful to say, "The cops have the guns. It's their problem; they can deal with it," (Deputy Chief M. Weir, Baltimore County Fire Depatrment, 9 May 2000). The complexity of these incidents makes it imperative that all emergency responders prepare, plan, and train for the time when violence explodes in the community.

Preparation

Preparation and planning are the keys to success in any disaster situation. The Tactical Emergency Medical Support Group of the Union County, New Jersey, Prosecutor's Office Emergency Response Team has conducted extensive preparations for such incidents at schools in their response district. Their activities can be used as a guideline for other EMS groups.

Box 15-1:   Mass-Casualty Shootings

Moses Lake, Washington February 2, 1996

Two students and a teacher were killed by a 14-year-old with a hunting rifle during an algebra class. Another student was left permanently injured.

Jackson, Mississippi April 24, 1996

After murdering his wife, a 32-year-old firefighter went on a shooting rampage in the central fire station killing five firefighters and wounding four others.

Pearl, Mississippi October 1, 1997

A 16-year-old stabbed his mother to death then proceeded to school with a hunting rifle. He killed two girls, one of whom was his former girlfriend, and wounded seven others.

Paducah, Kentucky December 1, 1997

A 14-year-old freshman with two shotguns and two .22-caliber rifles killed three students and wounded five others while the students were attending a prayer session in the hallway.

Jonesboro, Arkansas March 24, 1998

Two boys, aged 11 and 13, killed four girls and one teacher at their school. The boys were armed with three rifles, seven handguns, and 487 rounds of ammunition. Nine students and one teacher were also injured during the shooting.

Edinboro, Pennsylvania April 24, 1998

A 14-year-old boy killed a science teacher and wounded two students with a .25-caliber handgun registered to his father at an eighth grade dance.

Springfield, Oregon May 21, 1998

A 15-year-old freshman murdered his parents and then left for school armed with a .22-caliber semiautomatic rifle, a .38-caliber handgun, and military style knives. Two students at the school died and 23 people were injured. Two homemade explosives with electronic timing devices were later found in the 15-year-old's home.

Littleton, Colorado April 20, 1999

Two high school seniors heavily armed with both firearms and improvised explosives, killed 12 students and one teacher. Explosive devices were found planted in several areas of the school grounds. Over 160 people were triaged, 24 of whom had serious injuries. After their rampage, the two seniors took their own lives.

Conyers, Georgia May 20, 1999

A 15-year-old sophomore armed with a handgun and .22-caliber rifle wounded six students at Heritage High School.

Atlanta, Georgia July 29, 1999

During a rampage in an office building, a daytrader shot 21 people in an office building, killing nine. The bodies of his wife, son, and stepdaughter were found later at his apartment. When pulled over by police, the gunman killed himself.

Continued

Box 15-1: **Mass-Casualty Shootings** *Continued*

Los Angeles, California   August 10, 1999

A white supremacist attacked a Jewish Community Center, wounding three children, one teenager, and one adult. He later killed a postal worker while attempting to flee from police.

Fort Worth, Texas   September 15, 1999

A gunman walked into a Baptist Youth Rally and killed seven people and wounded seven others. He then killed himself.

Honolulu, Hawaii   November 2, 1999

A 40-year-old disgruntled Xerox employee killed seven colleagues with a 9-mm handgun. He surrendered after a five-hour standoff with police.

Seattle, Washington   November 3, 1999

A former employee of a shipyard returned with a gun and killed two men and wounded two others.

Tampa, Florida   December 30, 1999

A 36-year-old hotel employee shot and killed four coworkers. A fifth person was killed later by the same man during a carjacking.

Wilkinsburg, Pennsylvania   March 1, 2000

A gunman killed two men and wounded three others during a shooting spree in a suburb of Pittsburgh. The gunman later surrendered to police after a standoff in a building that housed both an adult and child daycare center.

Memphis, Tennessee   March 8, 2000

A firefighter killed his bride of three weeks and then set fire to her house. Two responding firefighters and one sheriff's deputy were killed by gunfire. A bystander was also wounded.

Wakefield, Massachusetts   December 26, 2000

An Edgewater Technology employee shot and killed seven co-workers after the IRS had his wages garnished for back taxes.

Melrose Park, Illinois   February 5, 2001

A former employee entered an engine plant and began to shoot. Four employees were killed and four others were wounded. After his rampage, the gunman took his own life.

Santee, California   March 5, 2001

A 15-year-old boy with a .22-caliber revolver killed two students and wounded 13 others at his high school.

El Cajon, California   March 22, 2001

Three students and two teachers were wounded by a shotgun blast at Granite Hills High School. The 18-year-old suspect engaged police in a running gun battle and was shot.

Grudy, Virginia   January 16, 2002

The Dean of the Appalachian School of Law, along with another professor and a student were shot and killed by a former student. The gunman had been dismissed for failing grades.

- Members of the group met with school officials to devise plans for meeting the challenges of a shooting on school property. This joint meeting ensured that everyone understood what steps would be taken and what information was necessary.
- They outlined vital information that would be needed in an emergency, including:
  - Detailed floor plans that showed the location of gas, electric, and water shut-off valves
  - Instructions on how to operate and silence any alarm systems (The police officers at Columbine High School were hampered by the loud noise of the building's alarm system.)
  - The location of any building communication systems or closed circuit television systems (CCTV) as well as instructions on how to operate them so that officers might track a suspect's movements and provide vital instructions to students and staff trapped in the building
  - Up-to-date copies of each school's standard operating procedures and emergency contact lists
  - Photographs of the school's interior and exterior, including aerial photos of the roof, to help familiarize police officers and other emergency responders with the structure's layout
- The assembled information, along with a complete set of building keys, is kept in the school office. In addition, all information was placed on a compact disc (CD) and stored at the command post so it could be readily accessed.

Most fire departments conduct pre-fire planning that targets hazards in their response districts. Because mass-casualty shootings occur at businesses as well as schools, these plans can easily be adapted to cover such incidents. Information such as building sketches, exit locations, alarm systems, and utility shut-off valves should already be part of these plans. The additional information noted above can be added to existing pre-fire plans with minimal effort. This is especially true if the agency uses a computerized pre-fire planning system. It may not be possible to develop pre-plans for every building and every type of possible emergency response, many of the hazards can be covered.

Plans for an incident at a school should take into account appropriate locations for triage, treatment, and transportation areas; helicopter landing zones, and the command post. Many schools are surrounded by open playing fields and parking lots, which may seem to be ideal locations for these areas. However, they also provide a wide field of fire, perhaps more than ½ mile around the school, which should be taken into consideration. If a triage area or command post is visible to the suspect, it may become a target. This will most certainly allow a chaotic situation to deteriorate even further. Additional information on mission planning can be found in Chapter 14, Tactical EMS.

Communications

Effective communications are crucial at major incidents and disasters. Obtaining and maintaining an efficient communications system at such incidents, however, is often challenging, especially when mutual aid is requested. Interoperable radio systems or regional mutual-aid radio frequencies can alleviate coordination problems with mutual-aid units.

The newer 800 MHz radio systems give incident commanders (IC) greater flexibility. Incident functions or operations can be grouped by communications needs. These clusters are known as talkgroups. At a mass casualty shooting incident, one talkgroup may consist of responding EMS units. As the incident grows in complexity, the IC might find it useful to place the triage area on a separate talkgroup. The transportation and staging areas may be placed on a third talkgroup. The command staff may also elect to initiate their own talkgroup—all without overloading the radio system.

Dividing communications along the lines of the incident command system can alleviate the radio congestion often seen at major incidents. However, such a configuration can become manpower intensive. Each talkgroup needs to be monitored at the command post. If too many units are spread across too many talkgroups, the incident commander may lose control of the incident.

Another problem often seen at emergency incidents is the inability of firefighters and emergency medical technicians to talk, via radio, to the police. Firefighters and emergency medical technicians should be able to contact the on-scene police officer and find out whether the area is safe to enter. In many jurisdictions, this information is radioed from the police officer to the police dispatcher, who then contacts the fire or EMS dispatcher, who then radios the message to the designated unit. Transferring information in this manner is both inefficient and time-consuming. Additionally, critical pieces of information may be inadvertently omitted by the dispatchers.

If your jurisdiction uses an 800-MHz radio system for all public safety functions, a combined police/fire/EMS talkgroup can be established, like the "Talkgroup 99" used in Baltimore County, Maryland. Police and fire department units, whether mobile or portable can select "Talkgroup 99" when the need arises. If an officer needs a report number from Medic 1 for an earlier vehicle accident, both units can converse through this talkgroup. If both police and EMS units have responded to a mass-casualty shooting at an area mall, arriving officers can advise staged EMS units when the scene is secured and provide other information, such as the number of victims or floor location.

Command

The incident commander at such a scene has one goal: to save lives. Two initial strategies will accomplish that goal. First, stop the shooter (**Figure 15-1**). Police will need to ascertain whether the shooter is still on the scene and trying to kill people. If the suspect is still shooting, police will need to confine or place him in custody before the second strategy, treatment and transportation of the injured, can be implemented.

The success or failure of the operation will hinge upon cooperation between the command officers from both the police department and the fire/EMS agency. This is no time for egos to replace sound judgement. Neither agency is more important at this type of incident. Without

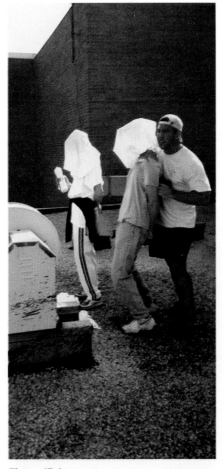

Figure 15-1 The active shooter must be stopped in order for EMS to begin caring for the injured. *(Courtesy Union County Emergency Response Team, NJ)*

coordination and cooperation between both agencies, the operation will be doomed to fail. A unified command is required, and high-ranking officials from law enforcement, fire, and/or EMS will need to assemble at a joint command post to manage the incident. It is counterproductive for the police command post to be on one side of the incident and the fire and/or EMS command on the opposite side of the incident. Command officers from all responding agencies must quickly be able to meet face-to-face to solve problems and implement necessary tactics.

Operations

As with any other shooting or stabbing incident, responding fire and EMS units should remain in the staging area until the scene is secured by law enforcement. If rescuers enter an area where a gunman is still loose, the rescuers can be injured by gunfire. Additional resources must then be used to extract and treat the firefighter or EMT. Remember, rescuers are there to be part of the solution, not part of the problem. As noted earlier, staging, treatment, and triage areas may need to be ½ to 1 mile away from the actual scene, depending on the geography around the building (**Figure 15-2**).

Another reason for keeping fire and rescue personnel in the staging area is the possibility that the suspect(s) may have planted explosive devices and other booby traps. At Columbine High School, nearly 100 explosive and incendiary devices were used.[1] One explosive device, placed approximately 3 miles from the school, was used to divert emergency personnel away from the action.[2] A planned attack at a community college in Cupertino, California, in January 2001 could have had similar results. A 19-year-old man was arrested only hours before the intended attack. Police found 30 pipe bombs, 20 Molotov cocktails, and several weapons.[3]

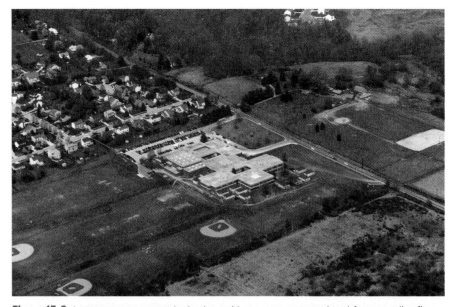

Figure 15-2 Large open areas around schools provide no cover or concealment for responding firefighters and emergency medical technicians.

Any information gained at the scene in the initial minutes should immediately be relayed to the incident commander. Often, emergency personnel responding to these situations encounter people fleeing the building. Although these people may be distraught, they can also be excellent sources of information. Can they describe the suspect(s), including height, weight, clothing? Where is the suspect located in the building? What type and number of weapons are being used? How many people are injured? Each piece of information is critical as the incident commander formulates an operational plan.

If SWAT-trained paramedics are used, they can handle this type of situation (**Figure 15-3**). The SWAT medics can enter with the SWAT/tactical team while the building is being secured and act as the eyes and ears of the command post, providing vital information that will allow the IC to call for additional resources in a more timely manner. As the SWAT medics move through the building, they can update the IC on the number of victims and their locations in the building. They can also provide information on the severity of injuries.

As the SWAT medic moves through the building with the tactical forces, he may have time to begin triaging patients. The simple act of tying red, green, or yellow ribbons on patients can save valuable time. However, it is the SWAT team leader, not the medic, who makes the decision about treating or moving on. If the team leader elects to move quickly to the area where the shooter is located, triage will have to wait. Remember, the first objective is to stop the violent actions of the person with the weapon.

Medics can also provide direction to civilians. If people are trapped in offices or classrooms, the medic can provide medical direction that may save the life of an injured person. The simple act of tilting the head back can clear an airway. Directing a student to place a towel over a bleeding wound and apply direct pressure can have significant results. Only lifesaving interventions should be applied until the patient is moved to a secure area. If people can leave the building through safe corridors, the medic may also direct workers or students to carry the injured out with them.

Many law enforcement agencies now use the term "active shooter" to describe a mass casualty shooting at a school or business. Since the deadly incident at Columbine High School, some law enforcement agencies are also re-thinking their approach to such situations. Many of these incidents occur quickly. Police may not have the time to secure a perimeter and wait for a SWAT team to assemble. These agencies have begun training their patrol officers to form a five-man team to enter the building before more specially trained forces arrive. The team attempts to locate and subdue the suspect(s), or limit the ability to inflict further casualties. This may mean confining the person to a room or area and waiting for assistance to take the person into custody.

This approach may allow more aggressive attempts by fire and EMS to retrieve injured civilians. If police can quickly enter and confine the suspect to a small area, firefighters and emergency medical technicians may be able to enter from a remote portion of the building to begin the processes of triage and transport. For example, if the suspect is confined

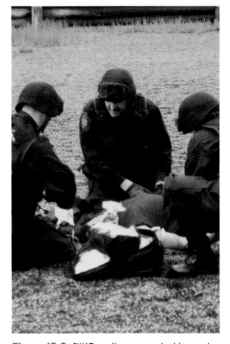

Figure 15-3 SWAT medics are a valuable asset at the scene of an active shooter. *(Courtesy Union County Emergency Response Team)*

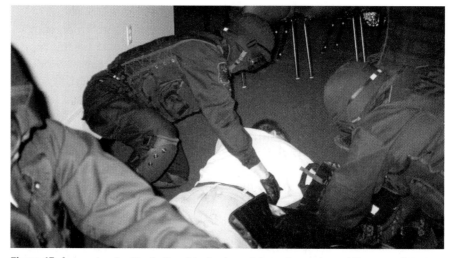

Figure 15-4 Agencies should not attempt to develop policies and procedures at the scene of a mass-casualty shooting. Fire/EMS and law enforcement must conduct joint training exercises to prepare for the active shooter incident. *(Courtesy Union County Emergency Response Team)*

to a classroom in the east wing of a school, safe entry might be possible on the far west side. Similarly, the rear loading dock of a business may be the entry if the shooter is cornered in a third floor front office. *However, such an operation should only be attempted when it is confirmed that all suspects are confined.* Only a small number of fire and/or EMS personnel should be allowed to enter the building under these circumstances. Additional police officers should also be entering the structure to ensure safe corridors for the removal of both unharmed and injured parties. As noted earlier, the healthy can help evacuate the walking wounded.

It is imperative that police and fire/rescue units conduct joint training sessions before these tactics are used at an actual incident (**Figure 15-4**). The site of a disaster is not the place to "try out" new ideas. If the security of fire and EMS personnel is ever in question, such tactics should not be employed.

SURVIVAL TIPS

1 Coordination and cooperation are the keys to success. Failure can mean the death of innocent civilians, police officers, firefighters, and emergency medical technicians.

2 Media access to this type of situation must be strictly controlled. Live video from the scene can warn suspects about the tactics being used by police and EMS personnel.

3 The suspect(s) may change clothes in an attempt to blend into the crowd. Police should clear all individuals leaving the building or area.

Chapter 16

Evidence Preservation

The increase in violent crime also increases the contact that emergency service providers have with the victims of crime. The EMS responder has a personal responsibility to ensure his or her personal safety, as well as a responsibility to the patient, whether victim or suspect, to provide emergency treatment and transportation to a medical facility, if appropriate.

In addition, the firefighter or emergency medical technician has a responsibility to the community at large. By assisting law enforcement to maintain the integrity of the crime scene, responders increase the probability that a suspect will be captured and convicted. That, in turn, reduces the possibility of future injury from additional crime.

Clearly, the first responsibility of the emergency medical responder, beyond that of personal safety, is to the patient. Preserving evidence at a crime scene must not take precedence over providing quality patient care. There are, however, simple techniques that can often accomplish both goals.

What Is Evidence?

There are a variety of definitions for the term evidence. *Black's Law Dictionary* defines evidence as "whatever is received to establish or disprove an alleged fact." A simpler definition useful for emergency responders is one provided by Donald W. MacKay of the Los Angeles City Fire Department. He states that evidence is "anything that a suspect has taken from, left at, or that may be otherwise connected with, the crime or crime scene." MacKay's definition is obviously concerned with things that can be sensed by touch, hearing, smell, taste, or sight.

Generally, there are two types of evidence: testimonial and real or physical. Testimonial evidence is the oral documentation by a witness of the facts.[1] Real or physical evidence is the critical link that ties a suspect or a victim to a crime. The objects left at the scene may prove a person innocent or guilty of a serious crime and may affect the lives of many people by the time the investigation is over. Evidence may provide the investigator with:

1. Proof that a crime has been committed
2. Proof that a given person was at the crime scene
3. The identity of a person(s) connected with the crime
4. The ability to exonerate an innocent person
5. Corroboration of the victim's story[2]

Physical evidence generally falls into three categories: body materials, objects, and impressions. Body materials include fluids and materials such as blood (either fresh or dried), semen, tissue, hair, earwax, and skin. Objects include weapons, soil, tools, and documents. Impressions are not feelings, but forms or figures left by physical contact. For example, a serologist can test body fluids and determine the person's blood type.[3] Biologic evidence can be genetically examined using the DNA molecule.[4] A single match lying beside a victim could be compared to the torn edges of a matchbook found in a suspect's pocket, linking him to the scene. The impression of a shoe print may link a suspect to a homicide or determine whether a driver had his foot on the brake pedal or the gas pedal at the time of an accident.

Critical Issues at Violent Crime Scenes

During violent crimes, minute particles called trace evidence will be transferred from the victim to the suspect and from the suspect to the victim. Trace evidence includes such items as hair follicles, clothing fibers, blood, semen, and saliva. If two people were struggling in a residence, there might be clothing fibers from each embedded in the carpeting or in the bedding. Hair might also be found on the claw of a hammer used to strike a person on the head. Although an investigator cannot state that hair from a crime scene specifically matches the hair of a particular person, the similarities between the two can be noted. For example, some of the information that can be determined from hair includes:

• Human or animal origin
• Race/sex
• Blood type
• Location on body: head, genital area, chest
• Whether the sample was pulled out, cut, fell out
• Whether the sample was dyed or bleached[5]

There might also be other types of trace evidence left at the scene including urine, feces, and even earwax. After a brutal attack, traces of skin might be found beneath the victim's fingernails. Pieces of tissue from either of the combatants might be found on clothing, on walls, or embedded in carpeting. Blood stains on walls, doors, clothing, or in carpeting also provide investigators with an array of information. Officials can tell the position of the victim in relation to the attacker, the type of weapon used, the number of blows or shots, and the movements of the victim and/or the assailant after the attack.

As a first responder or EMS staff, you must be concerned with your personal safety first. If you arrive on the scene of a shooting, stabbing, suicide, or similar incident, wait for law enforcement to secure the area before you enter. Follow police direction if you are asked to park in a specific area. They may be attempting to safeguard imprints of tire or foot tracks. As you approach the house or crime scene, be mindful of bullet casings, weapons, blood spatter, or puddles (**Figure 16-1**). Whenever possible, walk around such evidence. The police may have a clear pathway void of evidence that you can use. All crew members should use the same route to access the patient and to leave the scene. Any nonessential personnel should remain outside of the crime scene until needed.

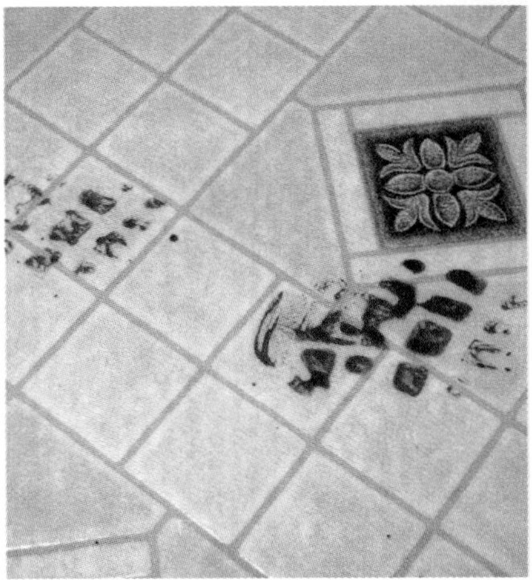

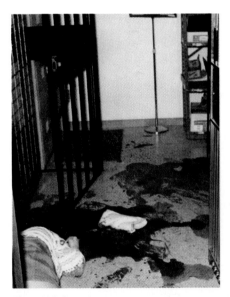

Figure 16-1 Evidence such as this bloody footprint can easily be destroyed by emergency responders entering crime scene.

When you open doors at a possible crime scene, try to use your shoulder, elbow, or the back of a hand. Even though you may be wearing gloves, grabbing a door knob with your hand could destroy any fingerprints on the knob. Once inside the scene, try to disturb as little as possible (**Figure 16-2**). Size up the scene as you would at a fire. Is the door open or closed? Are the lights on or off? If you arrive at an unknown crime scene before law enforcement, you may need to document these critical points.

Many departments use instant cameras to document the mechanism of injury at motor vehicle accidents. The photos are transported with the patient to the trauma center where surgeons can see the damage to the vehicle and plan subsequent treatment appropriately. Using a camera at a crime scene may be just as helpful. Certainly, if police are on the scene, they should handle these responsibilities. But if the first responding police officers do not have access to photographic equipment or if you unknowingly enter a crime scene, taking a few quick photos of the area may alleviate later problems for investigators. Remember, however, that patient care is more important than obtaining photos.

Continue the scene size-up by looking for any nearby weapons. Police should secure these objects if they pose a threat. If the patient is unconscious or deceased, the police may decide to leave the knife or gun in place for later photographic documentation and testing. Whenever you are treating a conscious patient, however, your safety is paramount and the weapon should be secured.

At the patient's side, perform an initial assessment. If the person is obviously deceased, try to alter the scene and the body as little as possible. If you begin treatment, be sure to put all dressing packages, medication packages, scraps of tape, and other extraneous materials in a biohazard bag and take it with you from the scene. If an object inadvertently falls to the floor, leave the object and note it to the police. Leaving medical items at the scene of a crime can complicate an investigation. Syringes found on the floor can point an investigation in a misleading direction. Latex or vinyl gloves at the scene may have been left by a criminal or by

Figure 16-2 Photo of actual crime scene.

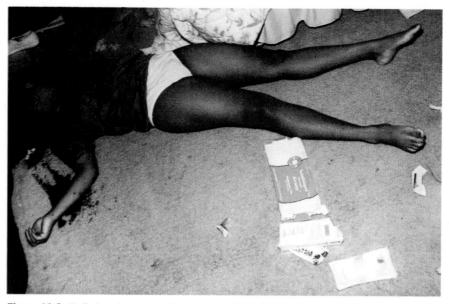

Figure 16-3 Medical waste can complicate a criminal investigation. *(Courtesy Baltimore County Police Department, Baltimore, MD)*

the responding emergency medical technician. The police and laboratory personnel may waste valuable time attempting to retrieve prints from the inside of discarded gloves left by responders (**Figure 16-3**). Do not pick up expended cartridge casings to determine the caliber. These fired casings may have fingerprints that could identify the criminal.[6]

Wound Ballistics

Ballistics is the study of the firing, flight, and effect of ammunition. You should understand the basic concepts that follow so you can properly preserve evidence at the scene of a crime or violent incident.

When a gun is fired, four things occur:

1. Flame is emitted from the barrel of the weapon.
2. Smoke is discharged behind the flame.
3. The projectile is discharged from the barrel of the gun.
4. Both burned and unburned gunpowder is discharged along with additional smoke.[7]

When a bullet strikes the skin, it causes an indentation and eventually perforates the skin surface. The reddish abraded area adjacent to the entrance hole is known as an abrasion collar.[8] As the bullet passes into the body, the skin returns to its normal position. Medical personnel should not guess the caliber of weapon used in an attack by the size of the gunshot hole, because the wound is typically smaller than the size of the projectile.[9] For example, in looking at a wound, emergency medical technicians may assume that a .22-caliber handgun was used when the actual bullet came from a .38-caliber weapon.

Gunshot wounds can also be categorized as contact, near contact, intermediate, and distant. Contact wounds can further be divided into hard, loose, or angled. A hard contact wound occurs when the muzzle of a gun is pushed tightly against the skin. The direct contact of the muzzle will cause charring to the edges of the wound. In addition, there will be a deposit of blackened soot directly adjacent to the hole (**Figure 16-4**). In a hard contact wound, the size of the hole will be larger than the size of the round. If the wound is over bone or skull, it may have a star-shaped pattern, also known as stellate.[10] If the firearm is not held tightly against the skin, a gap can occur between the barrel and the skin when the weapon is fired, causing a loose contact wound. In this case, a band of soot, known as smudge, may be deposited around the hole. If the weapon is not held perpendicular to the surface of the skin, the gap may exist only on one side, producing an angled wound. When the weapon is fired, hot air and soot may escape through this gap. The result will be a pear- or oval-shaped blackened zone to one side of the wound, generally opposite from the direction of the muzzle (**Figure 16-5**).[11] But investigators cannot automatically assume the direction of the muzzle merely by the placement of this pear-shaped stain. In near-contact wounds, this blackened area may lie on the same side of the wound as the muzzle of the weapon.

The intermediate-range wound is distinctive. When the weapon is held at least 10-mm away from the body, the burning powder and expelled fragments have a chance to disperse in a widening pattern.[12] They will produce reddish-brown hemorrhages known as tattooing or stippling when they strike the skin. The term *powder burns* should not be used to characterize any of the above conditions.

A distant gunshot wound, in which there is 18" or more from muzzle to target, will not display any tattooing, charring, or smudging.[13] There will, however, be an abrasion collar. The only distant gunshot wounds that will not have abrasion collars are those in the palms of the hands or the soles of the feet.[14] These wounds will be star-shaped.

Clothing

A variety of evidence can be found on the body of a shooting victim. But much of this evidence can be lost if responders are not careful. Trace evidence normally found on the skin of an exposed wound may also be embedded in clothing if the individual was dressed. Bullets may have traveled through the body but may not have exited the clothing. In blunt force injuries, an impression of the weapon used may also be left in the clothing.

When you remove clothes to expose a wound, do not cut through bullet holes, knife cuts, or tears (**Figure 16-6**). Once the clothes are removed, do not shake them because valuables, including valuable trace evidence, may fall from the pockets to the floor. In addition, trace evidence such as hair, can be anywhere on the clothes. Place each article of clothing in a separate bag. Even left and right shoes should be placed in separate bags. If both the victim and the suspect are at the scene and in need of medical attention, do not let their clothing come into contact with each other. If police are on the scene, merely remove clothing and place each article separately on the floor and notify officers of your actions. Stacking pants, shirt, underwear, and other items in one pile will cause cross-contamination of evidence.

Moist or wet evidence must be air dried. Critical evidence may be destroyed from the growth of microorganisms if moist or wet evidence

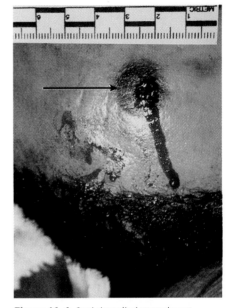

Figure 16-4 Soot deposited around near-contact wound. (*Courtesy Baltimore County Police Department, Baltimore, MD*)

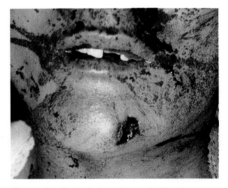

Figure 16-5 Oval-shaped wound. (*Courtesy Baltimore County Police Department, Baltimore, MD*)

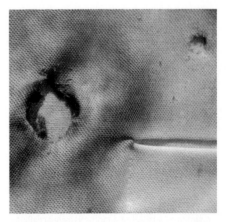

Figure 16-6 Burned and unburned gun powder, valuable evidence, may be deposited on clothing. Care should be taken in maintaining such evidence.

is left packaged for more than 2 hours. Paper bags are preferred over plastic bags because paper bags will not cause blood samples to degrade. If paper bags are not available, you may use biohazard bags, and transfer the evidence to paper bags as quickly as possible. If you collect any objects from the patient during transport or at the medical facility, notify police so that they can retrieve the evidence.

Sexual Assaults

Dealing with the victim of a sexual assault requires great care and consideration, particularly when treating the physical injuries. The patient has already experienced both physical and psychological trauma; the administration of medical services should inflict no further psychological damage. Investigating and prosecuting these crimes relies heavily on physical evidence.[15] For example, even a broken fingernail can be traced to a suspect months after the crime by comparing striations in the nail.[16] If the patient's condition warrants, wait for law enforcement to arrive and give you direction on what materials may be significant as evidence. Because seminal fluid may begin to break down due to drainage, enzyme activity, and other body acids, responders in rural areas may need to begin transport to a medical facility before police arrive.

The patient may feel compelled to wash or bathe, to change clothes, and to clean up the scene. But such actions destroy valuable evidence; encourage the patient to wait until the police arrive. If you must remove any clothing to provide care, bag each article separately, preferably in paper bags. Because bite marks may contain dried saliva, do not clean bite wounds with peroxide or any other antiseptic. Do not allow the victim to eat or drink until a physician takes oral samples.

Critical Issues at Vehicular and Pedestrian Accidents

Safeguarding and maintaining evidence at a serious motor vehicle accident are often overlooked by rescuers. Yet the scene may hold many clues for investigators. That is, of course, until rescuers spread a thick layer of absorbent material around to mitigate environmental hazards and then sweep up both the absorbent material and all the evidence that may have been present. Before you move or remove any object, whether it is a bumper or shard of glass, ask investigators whether it is appropriate to do so. Naturally, this action should not preclude patient care.

Once again, clothing can be significant to an investigator's case. When a motor vehicle strikes a pedestrian, the person's clothing may leave an imprint on the vehicle (**Figure 16-7**). Do not discard clothing, even at simple accidents.[17] The patient's clothing may contain minute chips of paint or glass fragments from the suspect vehicle. As noted earlier, even the driver's shoes can be significant if the soles left an imprint on the brake or gas pedals.

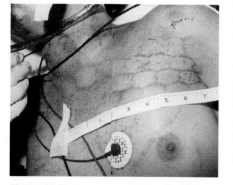

Figure 16-7 Bruising in the pattern of a tire left on victim as a result of a motor vehicle accident. *(Courtesy Baltimore County Police Department)*

Documentation

Frequently, fire and EMS personnel are called to give testimonial evidence in court and answer questions about what they saw or heard at the crime scene. In an area with a high call volume, this may be difficult unless the incident was properly documented. In many situations, a case may not come to trial for a year or more. Attempting to rely on memory alone is unprofessional and may even be embarrassing. Attorneys look for inconsistencies in witnesses' statements and attempt to discredit their testimony. Although some EMS personnel may think they can avoid court by not writing a complete report, this is simply not the case.

Three elements require proper documentation: what you saw; what you heard; and the chain of custody. When documenting your response to a crime scene, be as thorough as possible and provide a complete picture of the scene. Did you arrive before law enforcement arrived? If so, your description will be even more significant. How many victims were at the scene? Was anyone other than the police at the scene when you arrived? Were any characteristics of the scene noteworthy? Were the windows open or closed? Was the house ransacked? Were there any particular odors present, such as cigar or cigarette smoke, cleaning fluids, or fuel smells? Was the patient sitting or lying down? Face up or face down? Dressed or undressed?

Be as precise as possible in describing wounds without assuming anything. For example, write "single gunshot wound noted on left side of head above ear; tattooing and soot also noted around wound" rather than "tattooing and soot noted around wound on left side of head above ear, caused by a gun shot from 11" from victim's head." Do not draw conclusions or overstate the facts. Leave such assumptions to criminal investigators.

You should also note any statements made by the patient during transfer to the medical facility. Although you should not attempt to interrogate the patient, he or she may volunteer information that could later prove to be critical to the investigation. Anything that is freely stated and pertinent to an investigation should be noted. For example, if your patient was struck by a motor vehicle and begins to describe the car, it would certainly be appropriate to document the information and forward it to police when you arrive at the hospital. Or perhaps your patient, with no coercion, begins to brag about the gun battle in which he was wounded. Many jurisdictions require that a police officer accompany the patient to the hospital. If law enforcement is not on the scene or if they do not have sufficient manpower to accompany you, documenting such statements will be your responsibility.

Finally, your report should reflect any evidence found on the patient. Courts require the prosecutor to show that the evidence collected at the crime scene is the same evidence being presented in court. This chain of custody ensures that the evidence was not contaminated or tampered with. Law enforcement must be able to prove who handled a piece of evidence and when. In addition, they must show how evidence was altered as, for example, when blood found at a scene is tested. Each person who handles a piece of evidence must be noted on the tag that accompanies the evidence package. If the court finds a breach in the chain of custody, particular aspects of a case may not be admissible. For instance, as you transport a patient with a gunshot wound to the hospital, you begin to remove the person's clothes. You do not realize that the bullet is caught in the patient's down jacket. When you arrive at the hospital, you take the patient into the emergency department. After you complete your report, you return to your unit to retrieve the clothing. But because the jacket was left unattended and in the rear of an open ambulance, it may be difficult for prosecutors to have the bullet admitted as evidence.

Whenever possible, police should take immediate custody of any evidence. If you find evidence on your patient, note what was found in your report. Provide a description of each article and state who took custody of the item(s).

SURVIVAL TIPS

1. Do not wash your hands at the crime scene. Trace evidence such as hair may be in the sink and associated plumbing. Any evidence will be lost by running water into the basin.

2. Do not use towels at the scene to wipe up blood. Blood spatter and pooling provide valuable clues for investigators. The towels themselves may contain trace evidence that will be destroyed if they are used.

3. Urine sample containers may be used to collect bullet fragments, casings, or other small pieces of evidence found on your patient. Remember, each fragment or casing must be maintained in a separate container to prevent cross-contamination.

4. Telephone receivers may contain trace evidence such as fingerprints, earwax, or saliva, and should not be used. In addition, police can trace the last telephone call by using the *69 feature; if you use the phone, this trace will be misleading.

5. On critical incidents, police should accompany you to the hospital.

6. If your patient is tied with rope or some other type of binding, do not untie the knots. Cut through the material at a point distant from the knot. Segregate and bag the binding material.

7. If a patient is bound with duct tape, do not crumple the tape and discard after removal. Police can freeze the tape and pull apart each layer. The tape can then be checked for fingerprints.

Chapter 17

Gangs

*G*angs *pose an increasing threat in communities across the nation. This chapter is designed to raise your level of concern when you respond to areas where gangs are located, as well as help you to identify areas where gang activity is present or beginning to take root. Although it includes some survival tactics that can be used during gang-related incidents, most of the survival strategies described throughout this text can be adapted and used.*

The gang problem in the United States is not new. Ethnic gangs have been a problem for urban law enforcement since the turn of the twentieth century. Researchers at the University of Chicago who studied gang activity in 1927 found 1,313 different gangs in Chicago.[1] Outlaw motorcycle gangs began to emerge shortly after World War II. In the 1970s, little attention was paid to gangs, although at least one study suggested that gang violence was more prevalent than ever. The Vietnam War, the civil rights movement, and subsequent riots diverted attention by the media and public away from the gang problem.[2] Gang activities rebounded in the 1980s. What was once only a problem in major cities such as New York, Chicago, and Los Angeles is now a problem being experienced by smaller suburban and rural communities. In 1980, there were 2,000 gangs with 100,000 members in 286 jurisdictions; by 1996, the number had grown to approximately 31,000 gangs with over 846,000 members in 4,800 jurisdictions.[3] The latest statistics available show a slight decrease: 28,700 gangs and 780,200 gang members in 4,463 jurisdictions.[4]

The Hollywood portrayal of gangs and media attention to the youth problem have given many of these groups a mystique that youngsters may initially find attractive. For example, football players Charles Jordan and Chris Mims, as well as basketball star Stacey Augman, all admitted to gang affiliations. Jordan has even been seen to use gang hand signs during televised games.[5]

The idea that gangs are comprised of inner-city kids, are well-organized, heavily involved in the drug trade, and very dangerous is only partly true.[6] Although this may describe gangs in some communities, gang violence now reaches many suburban and rural areas. A recent survey noted that 81% of suburban counties with populations of 250,000 or more report problems with youth gangs. Similar problems are reported by 21% of rural counties with fewer than 100,000 residents.[7] Although the gang problem in Los Angeles, where 1 of every 100 residents is a gang member, is highly publicized, you may not realize that a similar situation exists in Albuquerque, New Mexico, where 1 of every 65 residents is a gang member.[8] Gangs are also a powerful presence in prisons; 54% of inmates in Illinois state prisons are gang members.[9] Super gangs are expanding their territories outside of their home states. The Bureau of Alcohol, Tobacco, and Firearms reports that in 1991, the Crips and the Bloods, two gangs that began in California, had sets operating in 32 states and 69 cities outside of the state.[10]

Youths generally join gangs for the following reasons:

- Identity
- Discipline
- Recognition
- Love
- Belonging
- Money

If you believe that gangs are strictly an urban problem, you may be vulnerable to unexpected youth violence in suburban neighborhoods. Firefighters and emergency medical technicians should be able to recognize the signs of gang infiltration. Once, spray painting walls in a back alley or on the rear of a shopping center was considered an adolescent prank; now, it is a sign of an impending problem, one that might prove dangerous to emergency responders (**Figure 17-1**).

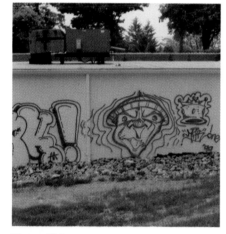

Figure 17-1 Back alleys are targets for graffiti and may hold clues to gang infiltration.

What Is a Gang?

One of the problems experienced by officials is the question of how to define a gang. Researchers use a variety of definitions when studying the gang problem. For instance, some researchers believe there is a difference between drug gangs and street gangs, while others draw no such distinctions. Motorcycle gangs, prison-based gangs, graffiti taggers, and racial supremacist groups may or may not be considered as gangs.[11] There is no legal meaning for the term "gang." The Federal Bureau of Investigation defines a gang as "a group of three or more individuals bonded together by race, national origin, culture, or territory, who associate on a continual basis for the purpose of committing criminal acts."[12]

Another problem is the widespread denial that gangs exist in an area. Law enforcement officials, school administrators, and even elected officials will routinely deny that their communities are experiencing gang problems. In one instance, EMS personnel questioned a county executive about an increasing problem with gangs within their jurisdiction.

The official vehemently denied that gangs were operating in the area and discontinued any further discussion on the matter, even though graffiti from a variety of gangs—including the Crips—had been noted. Naturally, denying that there is a problem effectively prevents finding a solution.

Some gangs are even becoming involved in local politics, with gang members running for office. In 1995, Wallace "Gator" Bradley, of the Black Gangster Disciples, ran for a seat on the Chicago City Council. Bradley's unsuccessful campaign was backed by the political arm of the Black Gangster Disciples known as 21st Century VOTE.[13] The Black Gangster Disciples have also been linked to the Save the Children Foundation.[14] The authors of *Gangs: A Handbook for Community Awareness* write:

> "The rash of much-publicized gang truces and peace summits are directly related to the political ambitions of street gangs. Many of these peace negotiations appear to provide hope for an end to street gang warfare. The reality centers on the mutual benefit that street gangs and politicians gain through each other. The street gangs gain positive recognition and achieve political legitimacy when they participate in these events. They can then manipulate community leaders and further increase their own power and influence. Using the cover of their peaceful activities in promoting a truce, a gang can continue to operate with less pressure. Politicians, eager to look good, order police to ease up on the gangs in order to ensure continued cooperation. The 'cooperating' gangs can then use the legitimacy and free publicity to build up membership and eliminate rivals during the truce."[15]

The authors also note that such political posturing has been effective in obtaining large sums of local, state, and federal monies earmarked for job training, recreation, education, and housing, and diverting them to purchase guns and drugs for gangs.[16]

Gangs are also attempting to infiltrate various government agencies such as the court systems and correctional systems. In some states, gangs have virtually taken over the prison system. Within prisons, gang members control the distribution of drugs and weapons and, in some cases, they also control food distribution as well.[17] Even the armed forces are experiencing problems with gang members infiltrating the military. Two uniformed members of the National Guard with Molotov cocktails in the trunk of their personal vehicles were arrested during the civil disturbances in Los Angeles in 1992.[18] Gangs have also attempted to acquire military weapons and explosives.

Gang Structure

All gangs are not the same. They wear different clothing of varying colors and styles to display loyalty to their group. They use hand signs to display affiliations with some groups and use sophisticated ciphers and code words to pass information between members (**Figure 17-2**). But

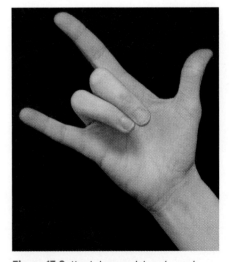

Figure 17-2 Hand signs are integral—each group has their own hand sign.

the differences between gangs goes beyond the mere physical attributes of clothing, hand signs, tattoos, and monikers. Gangs may be either loosely organized or have a more structured organization with formal leadership roles such as president or boss. Some gangs such as the Latin Kings have even held national meetings.[19] As noted in *Gangs: A Handbook for Community Awareness,* gangs evolve on a continual basis with structures and leaders changing constantly. Members appear, disappear, and reappear at a later date. What may initially appear to be kids spray painting a wall with unknown designs may quickly develop into a territorial gang that participates in drug dealing and violence. Gangs themselves may even disappear or reorganize. For instance, in 1982, a Detroit gang known as Young Boys Incorporated, which reportedly made $7.5 million a week and over $40 million annually, was targeted by federal law enforcement and dismantled.[20]

Some street gangs are strictly controlled by their prison gang counterparts. In 1993, there was a 15% drop in Latino gang-related murders after the Mexican Mafia prison gang decreed that drive-by shootings involving Latino street gangs should cease. The decree was made because violence among gangs was having a negative impact on the Mexican Mafia's drug trade.

Law enforcement uses three basic classifications to categorize gangs: territorial, corporate, and scavenger.

Territorial. This type of gang, as it suggests, claims a geographical area. This area may be a shopping center where the group congregates. It may be an apartment complex where most of its members reside or it may be an entire community. The group attempts to control all criminal activity in their "hood" or "barrio."

Corporate. The sole purpose of this type of gang is to make money. They will use whatever means available, including violence, to improve profits. Corporate gangs often begin as territorial groups. After taking control of more and more "turf," the organization looks more like a business than a loose group of violent kids.

Scavenger. Members of this type of gang have an overwhelming need to belong to a group. There is little organizational structure and most crimes committed by the group are on a spur-of-the-moment basis.

There are also different levels of gang membership, including:

Hardcore Members. These members build their lives around the gang and its activities. They wear the clothing, "throw" the hand signs, and commit the crimes necessary for the organization to survive. Their allegiance to the group is unwavering.

Fringe Members. These people want the emotional ties provided by gang involvement. Although they may wear the attire and throw the hand signs, they usually do not become involved in the more violent criminal activity seen with hardcore members.

Wannabees. School systems often feel that children who wear gang apparel and use gang signs are merely imitating gang members and are not a specific threat. Given the opportunity, these wannabees may join a local gang.

Gang members often operate on what might be considered their own "three R's:" reputation, respect, and retaliation. Reputation provides status for individuals as well as the gang itself, and is gained through the commission of crimes. Closely associated to reputation is respect, which may actually be fear. The thought of gaining respect from peers is a common force that drives adolescents to gangs. Respect and reputation are often gained by spending time in jail. A common tactic is to disrespect or "dis" rival gangs and gang members. This can be accomplished simply by throwing gang hand signs in a rival's territory. Such disrespect will normally lead to the third "R," retaliation. To maintain their respect and reputation, a gang or individual gang member must retaliate whenever "dissed." Such retaliatory acts are normally violent.[21]

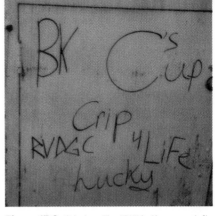

Figure 17-3 Crip tag. The "BK" in the upper left corner stands for "blood killer." *(Courtesy Sergeant John Marsh, United States Park Police)*

Specific Groups

West Coast Gangs. One of the greatest myths about gangs is that there are only two major rivals—the Crips and the Bloods. In the Los Angeles area, there are hundreds of gangs. Although independent of each other, most of these gangs, or sets, are aligned under either the Crips or the Bloods. There may be more than 120 Crip sets and more than 63 Blood sets in the Los Angeles area alone.

The Crip gang originated around 1970 at the Washington High School in Los Angeles (**Figure 17-3**). The name probably comes from the television horror show, "Tales of the Crypt." Initially, gang members were heavily involved in robbery and extortion at many school campuses. As their numbers grew, many gangs began to form alliances under the Crip umbrella. To combat the threat of the Crip gangs, the Bloods were formed. The Bloods originated in the early 1970s at Centennial High School in Compton, California, a suburb of Los Angeles. The original members, all from Piru Street in Compton, called themselves the Piru Street Boys.

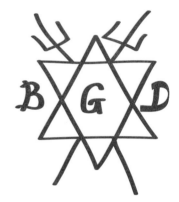

Figure 17-4 Black Gangster Disciples insignia. Each point of the star used by the Folk Nation has meaning: Life, Loyalty, Love, Wisdom, Knowledge, and Understanding.

Crips outnumber Bloods almost three to one. Thus, unlike television portrayals of fights between rival gangs, Crip sets fight amongst themselves more often than they fight with their sworn enemies, the Bloods. The Crips and the Bloods have become so powerful that they are spreading out from Los Angeles into cities across the nation.

Midwest Gangs. Chicago-based gangs are organized under the concept of nations. In 1979, the Black Gangster Disciples aligned with the Simon City Royals and approximately 20 other Chicago-area gangs to form the Folk Nation (**Figure 17-4**). The People Nation grew out of a gang known as the Blackstone Rangers, which, at that time, was run by Jeff Fort (**Figure 17-5**). The Vice Lords (rivals of the Black Gangster Disciples), the Latin Kings, and other gangs joined the People Nation

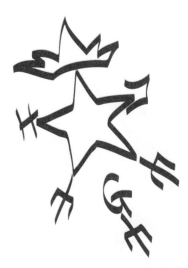

Figure 17-5 The People Nation uses a five-pointed star.

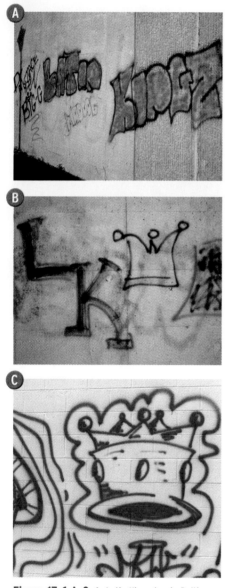

Figure 17-6 A–C A. Latin Kings tag in Baltimore County, MD. **B.** and **C.** The Kings will use either a three-pointed or five-pointed crown.

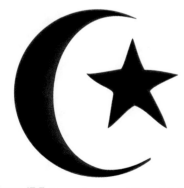

Figure 17-7 Crescent moon and five-pointed star used by the El Rukns.

(**Figure 17-6, A–C**).[22] Fort took the power of his gangs with him when he was sentenced to prison and established the El Rukns gang (**Figure 17-7**). This group was also aligned under the People Nation. In 1987, Fort and other El Rukn members were convicted of plotting terrorist activities with Muammar Qaddafi of Libya.[23] As with the Crips and Bloods, many of the gangs aligned under the Folk and People Nations are expanding into areas far removed from Chicago, including Florida, Georgia, Connecticut, and other states.

Hispanic Gangs. Hispanic gangs are turf-oriented. Even if a member moves away from his original area or barrio, he will always associate with the gang from his home neighborhood. Members might wear baggy khaki pants with white tank top t-shirts or Pendleton shirts and bandannas. Emergency responders should remember that to insult or "dis" an Hispanic gang member can be dangerous. Retribution may not always be immediate; however, to maintain status (save face), the member or gang will require some form of violent retribution. Hispanic gang members may have a tattoo of three dots, signifying "mi vida loca" or "my crazy life." Although such a tattoo can be found anywhere on the body, it is usually located on the hand, face, or neck. Many gang members, regardless of ethnicity or affiliation, will have a teardrop tattoo under one eye. Generally, this means that the member has spent time in jail.

The Mexican Mafia is a prison-based gang formed in the 1950s in the California Division of Corrections. However, their influence extends over many activities outside of prison. Like the historic Mafia gang, the Mexican Mafia is well organized and disciplined. They use killings to intimidate and to maintain discipline. Murders conducted by the Mexican Mafia may be very gruesome. The gang has also formed an alliance with the Aryan Brotherhood, and each group will honor the other's hit list.[24] The Mexican Mafia is also known as EME and Soreños.

In the 1960s, a group of Hispanic prisoners broke with the Mexican Mafia and formed La Nuestra Familia, or the LNF. Most of the members are rural farm laborers from northern California. Another gang, Northern Structure or Norteños, may be a subsidiary of LNF. Even though both the Mexican Mafia and La Nuestra Familia are considered prison gangs, many street gang members will identify with either Soreños or Norteños. Hispanic gangs from the Midwest or East Coast usually align with either the Folk Nation or the People Nation instead of with the Norteños or Soreños.

Note: Although non-Hispanics can become members of an Hispanic street gang, they may not always be accepted by their Hispanic prison-gang counterparts if they are arrested. Just as the Crips and Bloods do, the Norteños and Soreños are not only at war with each other but may also have disputes and wars with other sets within their family. Because the letter N is the fourteenth letter in the alphabet, members of Norteños will identify with the number 14. The Mexican Mafia and other Soreños will identify with the number 13. Both numbers will be used in graffiti, hand signs, and tattoos.

A relatively new gang is Mara Salvatrucha, which, loosely translated, means, "forever El Salvador." It is commonly referred to on the street as

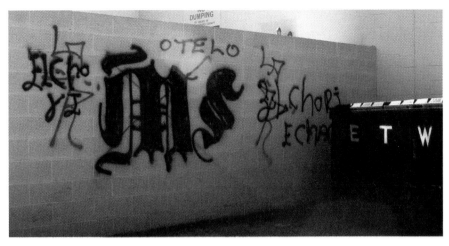

Figure 17-8 Mara Salvatrucha tag in Old English letters typical for many Hispanic gangs. The "MS" has been crossed out by a rival gang as a sign of disrespect.

"MS" or "MS 13." In the 1980s, Salvadorian refugees fleeing the civil war in their country began to settle in southern California and the Washington, DC, areas (**Figure 17-8**). Many of them had ties to violent street gangs and paramilitary groups from their homeland. MS was originally formed as protection against other Hispanic gangs in the Los Angeles area, but is now active in Alaska, Texas, Nevada, Oregon, Utah, Georgia, Michigan, New York, Maryland, and Florida. Although members are no longer strictly Salvadorian, they are predominantly of Central American ancestry. As with any other gang, MS participates in a wide range of criminal activities, including illegal military weapons sales, drug trafficking, extortion, rape, murder, auto theft, burglary, and witness intimidation. They show no fear of law enforcement and have killed three federal agents and shot many other police officers throughout the country.

Asian Gangs.   The history of Asian gangs dates back to 17th century China with the Triads, secret societies formed to fight unjust rulers and later became involved in criminal activities.[25] Chinese immigrants came to the United States as part of the labor force working on railroad construction and mining in the mid 1800s. The Chinese immigrants formed societies called Tongs to benefit the community, unfortunately, some of these societies also became involved in criminal activities.[26] Today, law enforcement is faced with the growing problem of several Asian gangs, including Cambodian, Korean, Filipino, and Laotian. All are somewhat secretive organizations,that are difficult to infiltrate.

Generally, Asian gangs focus their crimes against people of their own nationality, although recent evidence suggests that this is changing. Home invasion robberies are popular and brutal. It is not uncommon for the gang members to torture family members to force them to relinquish all valuables. Extorting businesses for protection money is also very popular. These gangs are also involved in credit card fraud, cellular phone cloning, and trafficking in stolen computer chips.

Due to their secretive nature, Asian gangs employ subtle means of identification. Historically, they have avoided the use of colored clothing

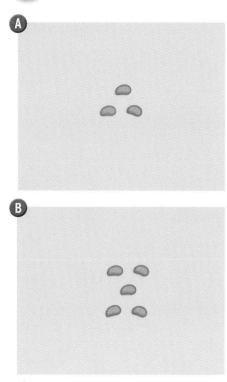

Figure 17-9 A and B A variety of burn marks or brands have subtle meaning within Asian gangs.

and large tattoos to show gang affiliation. The more subtle use of scars and burns has been the trademark of the Asian gang. For instance, a pattern of three (**Figure 17-9 A**) or five (**Figure 17-9 B**) burn marks on the hand might denote criminal activity; a scar in the form of "TRG" usually represents a group called "Tiny Rascals Gang."

Note: The series of three dots is also used by the Hispanic gang, 2-6 Nation, which is aligned with the Folk Nation. In this gang, the three dots stand for third world organization.

Motorcycle Gangs. Although small in number compared to street gangs like the Bloods, the Crips, or the Gangster Disciples, outlaw motorcycle gangs (OMG) are considered by law enforcement to be well-organized groups that rival the Mafia. Most law enforcement agencies point to a Fourth of July incident in 1947 as the catalyst that brought attention to OMGs. During a motorcycle rally in the small town of Hollister, California, two members of a motorcycle gang were arrested. The town was ravaged during the ensuing riot as other gang members attempted to gain freedom for their colleagues. A short time later, the first chapter of the Hell's Angels was established in San Bernadino, California (Krebs DR, Baltimore, MD, personal correspondence with Rachael Ridenour, 2001). Hollywood glamorized the bad-boy lifestyle of motorcycle gangs in the 1954 movie, "The Wild Ones," and in the 1969 feature, "Easy Rider." These films brought notoriety to the gangs and swelled their ranks. In response, the American Motorcycle Association noted that most motorcycle owners were law-abiding citizens and that only 1% were involved in criminal activity. Motorcycle gang members quickly adopted the term "1%er," proudly wearing patches emblazoned with the sign.

There are nearly 1,000 motorcycle gangs in the United States and Canada. The four largest are the Hell's Angels, the Bandidos, the Outlaws, and the Pagans. Many of these groups have chapters throughout the United States and around the world. Their criminal enterprises include bombings, arson, murder for hire, extortion, white slavery, money laundering, and gun running. Currently, their most lucrative enterprise is the distribution of methamphetamine. With the increasing popularity of this illegal substance, law enforcement is investigating relationships between OMGs and Mexican drug cartels that may be supplying large quantities of meth to the gangs for distribution throughout the United States.

Today's motorcycle gangs are highly organized. Most have by-laws and constitutions that govern the rights and obligations of members. Typically, these organizations have presidents, vice-presidents, and secretary-treasurers. In some gangs, an applicant is required to take a polygraph or voice stress analysis to ensure that the group is not infiltrated by law enforcement.

The Hell's Angels Motorcycle Corporation even has an Internet web site that markets clothing items displaying their trademarked "death-head" logo. The former leader of the Oakland chapter, Sonny Barger, even sells his own barbecue sauce. Reportedly, some gangs have formed "churches" and thus are eligible for local, state, and federal tax exemptions.[27]

OMGs remain dangerous. Many gang members are heavily armed and will quickly resort to violence. Some gang members have been known to rig shotgun rounds in the handlebars of their motorcycle, allowing them to shoot and possibly kill a police officer attempting a vehicle stop. Others find unique places to conceal edged weapons on their motorcycles. A popular trick is to weld a knife blade to the underside of the gas cap. The concealed knife can be easily reached by the rider.

White Supremacist Groups. White supremacist groups have post-Civil War origins, beginning with the formation of the Ku Klux Klan (KKK) (**Figure 17-10**). Many of these organizations operated covertly in their communities, often with the cooperation of the community. Until the Civil Rights movement, the often violent anti-Semitic and racially divisive activities of the KKK and other white supremacist groups were well-known but not widely publicized. Today, an increasing number of groups are continuing to spread a message of hate. The Aryan Nations, the Church of the Creator, and the Phineas Priesthood even attempt to link their social beliefs with religious beliefs and constitutional freedoms from religious persecution (**Figure 17-11**). In fact, many Neo-Nazi and white supremacist groups are aligning under the Christian Identity movement.

Skinheads, or White American Skin Heads (WASH), are considered part of the white supremacist movement (**Figure 17-12**). Their usual attire includes steel-toed Doc Martin boots, Red Tag Levis, suspenders (also called braces), and bomber jackets. Tattoos may include Nazi swastikas, lightning bolts, hammers, and Confederate flags. Like many other gangs, skinheads are beginning to use more subtle means of displaying their affiliation. For example, most emergency responders would not associate a tattoo of two eights (88) with skinheads or any other white supremacist group. But the eighth letter in the alphabet is H and, to these groups, the subtle underlying message of the tattoo is "Heil Hitler."

There are two types of skinheads. The first is the racist Neo-Nazi who believes in the purity of the white race and opposes Jews, homosexuals, and nonwhites. The second group is known as Skinheads

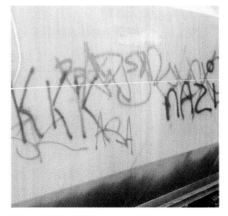

Figure 17-10 White supremacist groups are active in many parts of the country.

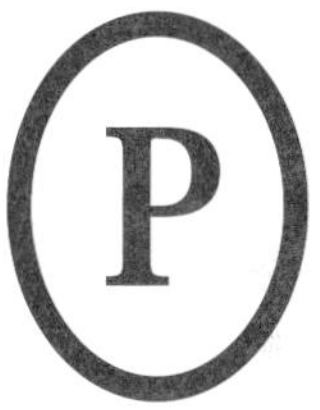

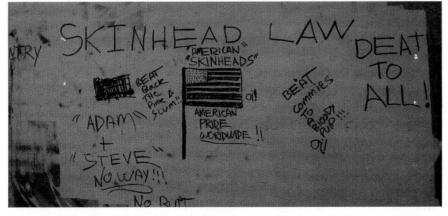

Figure 17-12 Skinheads are considered part of the white supremacist movement. (*Courtesy Sergeant John Marsh, United States Park Police*)

Figure 17-11 Phineas Priesthood members may wear items of clothing or tattoos with a "P" in a circle.

Table 17-1 Gang Affiliations

Gang Name	Affiliation	Color	Side Orientation	Clothing	Identifiers
Bloods		Red		Calvin Klein clothing ("CK" stands for Crip Killer)	Five pointed star
Crips		Blue		British Knights shoes ("BK" stands for Blood Killer)	Six pointed star Replace letter "B" in conversations with the letter "C" to disrespect Bloods
Folk Nation			Right		Six pointed star Rabbit with right ear bent Pitch fork facing up
Black Disciples	Folk	Black and blue Silver or white	Right	Denver Broncos apparel (Reverse initials for "BD")	Six pointed star
Black Gangster Disciples	Folk	Black, blue, white, silver	Right	Detroit Lions, Detroit Tigers, NY Yankees apparel (Black, blue, and white colors) Los Angeles Dodgers ("D" for Disciples)	Six pointed star Pitchforks Hearts with pitchforks
Latin Disciples	Folk	Blue and black	Right		Heart with tail or devil with horns. Tattoos with initials MLD or FMLDN
People Nation			Left	Converse shoes (Logo has five pointed star)	Five pointed star Playboy bunny with left ear bent
Bishops	People Nation		Left		Gothic letter "B" Bishop's cross
Vice Lords	People Nation	Black, red, green, and gold	Left	UNLV apparel (Vice Lords Nation United) Chicago Bulls (Colors are red and black) Louis Vuitton caps (Initials "LV")	Crescent moon Pyramid Top hat
Latin Kings	People Nation	Gold and black	Left	Los Angeles Kings apparel (Kings)	Initials ALKN Five pointed crown
El Rukns	People Nation	Black, red, green, and gold	Left		Crescent moon Pyramid Number 7 in a circle

Continued

Table 17-1 Gang Affiliations *(Continued)*

Gang Name	Affiliation	Color	Side Orientation	Clothing	Identifiers
Tiny Rascals Gang		Blue or grey		Hats with letters "TRG"	
Norteños		Red		University of Nevada Las Vegas clothing (UNLV – Us Norteños Love Violence)	Color red only used outside of California. Identify with the number 14 (The letter *N* is the fourteenth letter in the alphabet.)
Soreños		Blue			Color blue is only used outside of California.
MS		Blue and white			Often use the number 13. Use the term "mi vida loca," or my crazy life.

Against Racial Prejudice (SHARP) and is against racism. Both groups, however, will resort to violence to obtain their goals. Because both groups dress alike in bomber jackets, boots, and braces, they should both be treated with caution by emergency responders.

Female Gang Members. Responders should not discount the role of women in gangs. Until recently, female gang members generally provided support to their male counterparts, perhaps by serving as the driver in a drive-by shooting or by holding guns or narcotics for the males in the gang. Increasingly, however, female gangs are forming. Although they may be affiliated with the Folk Nation, People Nation, Soreños, or Norteños, these female gangs operate in their own distinct area and commit their own crimes, including drive-by shootings, robberies, and narcotic distribution.

Gang Affiliations. **Table 17-1** lists a number of gangs and their affiliations. Certain identifiers, as well as colors and sports team clothing that may be used to show alliance to a certain gang, are also listed. Some gangs will orient their clothing to one side or the other to show their alliance. A member of the Vice Lords may wear the left pant leg rolled up or turn the brim of his baseball hat to the left. A member of the Black Gangster Disciples may have a tattoo on his right arm. Gang members affiliated with the Folk Nation may fold the tongue of their right-foot sneaker up and leave the left down, while a member of the People Nation will do the opposite to his shoes. The right or left orientation may, however, be as subtle as folding one's arms and leaning to the right or left, depending on the gang. Another subtle means of iden-

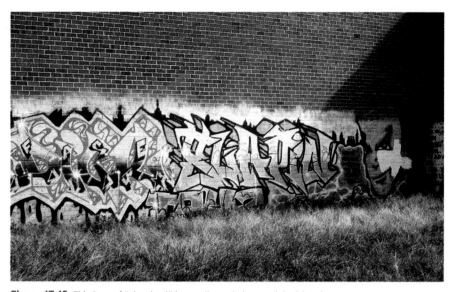

Figure 17-13 This type of "street art" is usually made by nonviolent tagging crews.

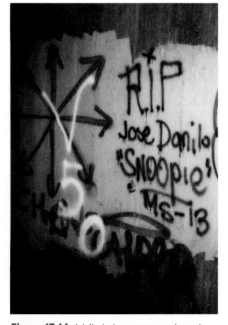

Figure 17-14 A tribute to a gang member, who had been killed, known as "Snoopie" from MS13. *(Courtesy Sergeant John Marsh, United States Park Police)*

tification is the use of military-style web belt. The brass buckle will be altered with initials, such as "TRG" for Tiny Rascals Gang.

Graffiti

Graffiti, or tags as they are known on the street, are an integral part of the gang culture. There are two types of graffiti that can be closely related. The often colorful artwork adorning many bridges, billboards, subway cars, and buildings is often viewed as a form of street art (**Figure 17-13**). The artist, more appropriately termed a tagger, attempts to place his or her renderings in as many places as possible. The risk of injury from scaling a bridge or crossing an energized third-rail of a subway line to spray paint a picture is considered a challenge. Such challenges enhance the celebrity status of the tagger. Other than the destruction of property, taggers, in and of themselves, do not represent a threat to the overall community.

Gang graffiti, however, have specific meanings and depict a threat to the community at large. These cryptic messages may signal a territorial claim, a message of condolence to a deceased member, or a challenge to another gang (**Figure 17-14**). Turf-oriented gangs will use graffiti to mark their territory and warn other gangs to stay away. If an opposing gang crosses out these territorial markers, the result is usually a violent confrontation. Another insulting tactic is to draw an opposing gang's insignia upside down. Asian gangs usually do not claim turf as many other gangs do, and they will merely place a tag near a local hangout.[28] Each gang and, more specifically, each set will use individualized tags in their territory. For instance, the Latin Kings in southern Florida may have somewhat different types of graffiti than the Latin Kings in Chicago. In general, graffiti from black gangs is usually less stylized than graffiti from Hispanic gangs. It takes very little training to enable firefighters and EMS personnel to decipher these tags and learn which gangs operate in their response areas.

Working in Gang Areas

As an emergency responder, you should be aware of the trends in your community. Talk to local law enforcement and develop a relationship with officers in your response area. Ask them to provide you with information on the crime issues in your community, including any gang problems. If necessary, explain your interest. Most police officers will gladly share information on gangs and various other problems, once they realize your safety is at stake.

Local law enforcement officials can also provide specific information on individual gangs and their habits. They will know what clothing styles are being used and what hand signs have particular meaning. For instance, if a member of the Latin Kings wipes his shirt, it could mean "wipe him out." But clothing styles, hand signs, and colors are not universal. A piece of clothing associated with the Black Gangster Disciples in Chicago may not be used by the Black Gangster Disciples in Connecticut. More importantly, a person wearing a sports team jacket or a red bandanna is not necessarily a gang member. Each person must be viewed as an individual. Is the person wearing gang attire? Is there a tattoo associated with a gang? Has the individual been seen throwing hand signs? Do not forget the obvious—does the person claim to be a gang member? Most gangs look unfavorably on members who deny membership in their group.

As you familiarize yourself with your response district, maintain a watchful eye for gang graffiti. Here again, the local police may be able to explain the meaning of otherwise unintelligible scribblings on a wall. Although you do not need to become a gang expert, you should be interested in what areas (housing projects, shopping centers, apartment complexes) are being claimed as gang territory. Graffiti may not always be obvious. The rear walls of shopping centers and office buildings may contain interesting tags. Bridge overpasses and hallways of apartment buildings are also favorite locations for gang graffiti.

The use of contact and cover, described in Chapter 8, is an appropriate tactic when you are in neighborhoods influenced by gangs. The gathering crowd at the scene of a stabbing or shooting may assume you are doing injury instead of providing care. Your precise, methodical actions may be viewed by some as being slow and uncaring. You may hear someone in the crowd say, "Why don't you quit playing and get him to the hospital?" If you do not remain aware of everything going on around you, you could be caught off-guard. The inexperienced emergency medical technician needs to focus all attention on the injuries; the experienced emergency medical technician knows that one person on the crew needs to focus on and read the crowd.

In some gang areas, especially where drive-by shootings are prevalent, crews should consider personal safety and limit the amount of medical care provided out in the open. After a drive-by shooting, the gang may return to the scene to ensure that the target is dead. If they seen an EMS responder holding an IV over the victim, they may shoot a second volley of gunfire. The result might be not only a dead victim but dead responders as well. Victims of drive-by shootings should be given minimal care outside and loaded into the unit as quickly as possible, so that treatment can be continued in a more secure area. In certain instances, it may be advisable for crews to obtain police escorts when they respond to gang strongholds. In some communities, fire and EMS apparatus will wait for a police escort, regardless of the type of call.

Finally, always use common sense when dealing with gangs. Attempting to act like a gang member by throwing hand signs or using slang terms is very dangerous. For example, arriving at an emergency scene and addressing an onlooker as "cuzz" may have tragic results if you are speaking to a member of a Blood set. Your attempt to be "cool" will certainly be viewed as a sign of disrespect. The result can be a retaliatory strike against you.

Terminology

Bank: To strike or beat

Crab: Disrespectful slang name for Crips, used by Blood gang members

Crew: An interchangeable term with set, posse, and mob; some East Coast and Midwest groups heavily involved in the drug trade may use this term in association with a neighborhood name as in "Lakebrook Crew." Some groups attempt to capture the violent reputation of the Jamaican groups by adding posse to their name. In an attempt to mimic organized crime families gangs may adopt the term *mob*.

Cuzz: Greeting between members of the Crips

Deuce-Five: .25-caliber handgun

Double-Deuce: .22-caliber handgun

5-0: Originated with the television show "Hawaii 5-0;" the term means police and is often used as a warning to other gang members that law enforcement is in the area.

Gat: Gun

LA Sag: Clothing style where pants are worn below the hips displaying cleavage of buttocks

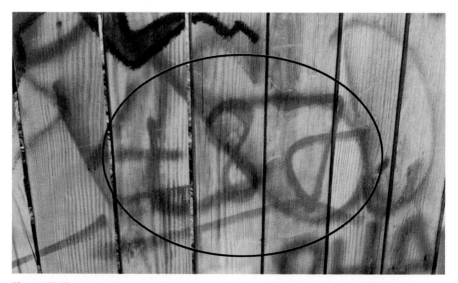

Figure 17-15 The use of *187* in graffiti is seen as far away as Washington, DC, and Baltimore, MD.

187: California penal code for homicide; this number will often be seen as graffiti and represents the group's willingness to kill (**Figure 17-15**).

211: California penal code for armed robbery

Moniker: Nickname given to a gang member by friends or family

OG: Original Gangster

Set: Subgroup of a particular black street gang; for instance, the Crips are said to have approximately 115 sets such as "59 Hoover," "Compton Crips," and "Eight Trey Gangster Crips." The term "clique" has a similar meaning in Hispanic gangs.

Slob: Slang name for Blood gang members and a means of disrespecting Blood members

Tool: Gun

Trey Eight: .38-caliber handgun

Varrio: Neighborhood

$: Power and money (**Figure 17-16**)

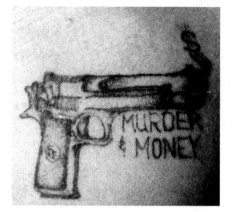

Figure 17-16 Tattoo on gang member's chest. The dollar sign in the smoke coming from the muzzle of the gun shows the youngster's two interests.

SURVIVAL TIPS

1. Tattoos are the most widely used method of identifying whether a person is a gang member.

2. The throwing of gang-type hand signs by fire and EMS personnel is unwise and can result in serious injury; some gangs may even kill a nonmember if that person is found wearing the gang's tattoo. Members of the deaf community have been beaten and shot when gang members misinterpreted their signing as disrespect.

3. Emergency responders should avoid addressing a gang member by his moniker. Use of these slang names by persons other than gang members is often perceived as disrespect.

4. When dealing with an injured member of a motorcycle gang, do not cut their "colors," the leather or jean jacket emblazoned with the gang logo. Members would rather endure the pain of moving a fractured arm than have their jacket cut.

5. Footwear is significant to both Skinheads and Hispanic gang members. As with cutting the colors of a motorcycle gang member, scuffing the shoes of a Skinhead or Hispanic gangbanger is seen as disrespect and can result in serious injury.

6. Skinheads may carry hammers stuffed down in their pants or have carpet knives in their back pockets.

Chapter 18

Less-Lethal Munitions

Police officers have a variety of nonlethal weapons at their disposal, including chemical sprays, bean-bag rounds, and rubber bullets. Firefighters and emergency medical technicians, particularly those who provide medical support to law enforcement SWAT teams, should be aware of these devices and the consequences of their use. That way, when you encounter them in the field, you will be prepared to deal with the emotional and physical results.

The Force Continuum

In recent years, law enforcement policies and procedures on using force have been criticized. As a result, police departments have reevaluated the techniques used to capture and subdue suspected criminals.

Most police departments teach their officers to use a "force continuum" to gain compliance. The "force continuum" is somewhat similar to the "continuum of care" treatment protocols used by many EMS systems throughout the country. In both situations, the least intrusive and most basic steps are taken first. If those steps are ineffective, progressively higher levels of intervention are used until the desired result is achieved.

For example, a paramedic would not defibrillate a person with 360 joules of energy if that patient was awake, responsive, and complaining of moderate chest pain. Instead, basic interventions, such as applying oxygen, would be used to alleviate the pain. Similarly, the law enforcement protocol begins with a basic intervention, the verbal challenge. The officer must tell the person what actions are expected, such as "put the knife down," "step back away from me," or "put your hands on the back of your head." If the person complies and follows the order, no further escalation of force is necessary.

However, if the basic intervention is ineffective, both the paramedic and the police officer must take additional steps to achieve their goals. In the case of the patient with chest pain, the paramedic might examine other variables, such as blood pressure, pulse, history, allergies, and ECG rhythm, before determining a course of treatment. Even while administering the treatment plan, the paramedic can apply other protocols if the steps being taken do not result in the desired outcome. Depending on the circumstances, the police officer may also proceed to other levels of force if the suspect does not comply with the verbal order.

The force continuum has several escalating levels that include pain compliance techniques and various physical strikes, such as those delivered with a baton. The use of chemical agents has had varying degrees of success. But until recently, the options from verbal order to physical confrontation to deadly force have been limited.

Today, many law enforcement agencies are employing "less lethal" kinetic energy impact projectiles to give officers more options in dealing with people.[1] For instance, a man threatening to commit suicide by shooting himself left few options open to law enforcement. Negotiators could attempt to talk the individual into giving up the weapon, or the police could shoot the person. The officer might not be shooting to kill, but simply trying to force the person to drop the weapon. Nevertheless, this alternative has become known as "suicide by cop." With the introduction of "less lethal" munitions, officers now have other tools to use in resolving such a situation.

Emergency responders should be aware that less-lethal munitions can cause injury and sometimes death. In the past 25 years, these devices have caused five deaths in the United States and Canada.[2] Emergency medical technician training provides little information on their specifications, deployment, and the injuries that can be expected. The remainder of this chapter will examine various chemical agents and munitions being used. Where possible, information was obtained from a variety of product manufacturers. Treating injuries from these agents and munitions should follow standard treatment protocols in your jurisdiction.

Tear Gas

The term "tear gas" has been widely used by the public for years. News reports show police using these chemical agents to disperse crowds during a civil disturbance or to flush out an individual who has barricaded himself in a structure. The use of chemical agents, however, is not new. As early as 2300 B.C., Chinese armies made "stink pots" by burning red pepper in hot oil to create an irritating smoke.[3] The ancient Greeks burned wax, pitch, and sulfur to create poisonous gases used in warfare.[4] Many of the current chemical warfare agents were developed during World War I. The first documented case of chemical agent use by law enforcement occurred in 1912 when the Paris police used a chemical (ethylbromacetate) that would cause a runny nose and tearing eyes.[5]

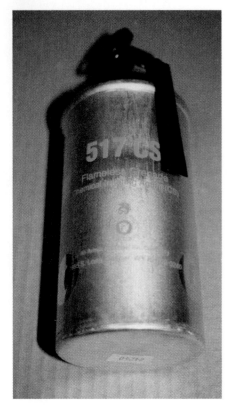

Figure 18-1 CS gas in a pyrotechnic delivery system.

Currently, there are three agents in general use: Chloroacetophenone (CN), orto-chlorobenzylidene-malononitrile (CS), and oleoresin capsicum (OC). Although CN and CS are commonly referred to as gases, these agents are actually micron-sized particles (1/25,000 of an inch), which can be delivered in a variety of ways.

- Pyrotechnic device: the chemical is mixed with other materials that burn in a grenade-type casing. The smoke emitted carries the chemical agent. As the name implies, pyrotechnic devices develop high temperatures and generally are not used indoors (**Figure 18-1**).
- Liquid: the chemical agent is suspended in a liquid that can be dispensed from either an impact projectile or an aerosol can. When the impact projectile strikes, it breaks open, splashing the liquid into the air as a mist. When contained in a sealed container and released under pressure, the mixture resembles hair spray or deodorant (**Figure 18-2**).
- Dust: the chemical agent is housed in a projectile as a fine dust. When the projectile strikes and breaks open, the dust is dispersed.[6]

CN was one of the initial "harassing agents," as they came to be known, developed in World War I. In its natural state, CN is a colorless crystalline substance at room temperature. It is a lacrimating agent and respiratory irritant. CN affects the lacrimal glands, causing heavy tearing, as well as coughing, sneezing, and a burning, runny nose. Both chest tightness and skin irritation might be noticed. The skin irritation may result from high temperatures and humidity, as well as from sweat and overexertion. Nausea and vomiting may also be present. A concentration of 35 mg/mv³ to 40 mg/mv³ can be toxic, and 1,000 mg/meter³ can be lethal. Five deaths have been reported after exposure to CN. In each of these cases, the subject was in an enclosed area.

Because CN is one of the products used in chemical mace, many people have the false impression that this agent will be useful against animals. However, most animals that do not have lacrimal glands, including dogs, perform well in the presence of either CN or CS.

CN is chemically unstable, which led military scientists to search for better agents. In 1928, B. B. Corson and R. W. Stoughton developed orto-chlorobenzylidene-malononitrile (CS), a white crystalline substance. However, the US military would not adopt its use until the early 1960s. CS is highly efficient and has almost totally replaced CN. It is also significantly safer, with a lethal dose at 6,000 mg/mv³.

CS has a pepper-like odor and produces symptoms similar to CN almost immediately upon exposure. Symptoms include burning of the eyes, nose, throat, and tongue; tightness in the chest; coughing; and shortness of breath. The nose will run, the eyes will involuntarily close, and the person may become agitated and begin to panic. As with CN, the skin may sting, especially in moist areas. Its effects last for approximately 5 to 10 minutes after the person is removed from the contaminated atmosphere.

Emergency care for both CN and CS exposure is relatively simple. The patients should be moved upwind and away from the contaminated area. They should face into the wind and keep their eyes open. They

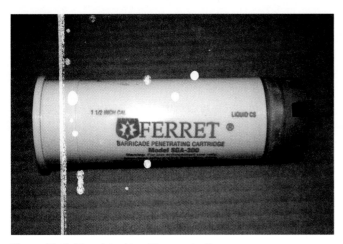

Figure 18-2 CS contained in a 37-mm projectile.

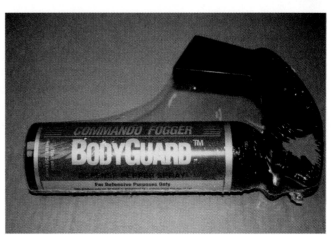

Figure 18-3 Oleoresin Capsicum (OC) Spray commonly called "pepper spray."

should avoid rubbing the eyes because this may force the particles further into the eyes. In some cases, the eyes and skin will need to be flushed with cool water. Most people will recover rapidly once removed from the area.

If further medical treatment is required, emergency responders should realize that chemical agents, especially CS, can pose difficulties during transport to a medical facility. Contaminated clothing should be removed and the skin flushed with water for 10 to 15 minutes before transporting the patient. If the patient is not adequately decontaminated before being placed in the transport unit, the crew may develop exposure symptoms themselves. In addition, bringing a contaminated patient to the al emergency department can quickly shut it down. If you must port a patient who has not been properly decontaminated, notif eceiving hospital of your situation. The hospital may request that y ke the patient to an alternate location, thus avoiding problems main emergency department.

OC Spray

Many law enforcement agencies across the country use the aerosol restraint spray oleoresin capsicum (OC) spray commonly called "pepper spray" (**Figure 18-3**). OC is a nonlethal aerosol that incapacitates with no lasting aftereffects. It can immobilize an attacking human or animal for up to 45 minutes. A derivative of cayenne peppers, OC is an inflammatory agent not an irritant. The capsicum (hot pepper) portion of the spray is suspended in a carrier, the oleo resin, which also allows the capsicum to adhere to the skin. All ingredients are approved by the Food and Drug Administration (FDA) for use in food and pharmaceutical. The propellant often used is a DuPont product called Dymel, which is nonflammable and noncarcinogenic.

A 1-second burst into a person's face will cause a loss of coordination, interrupt thought processes, and disrupt upper body control. This shoul capacitate the person and ensure compliance. The police officer m e additional sprays if the subject does not comply. OC spray causes inflammation of the mucous membranes in the eyes, nose, and throat. As the capillaries in the eyes dilate, the eyes will involuntarily close. The larynx is paralyzed, causing shortness in breath, coughing, and gagging, as well as nasal and sinus drainage. Blood vessels also dilate so there is increased blood flow to the affected area. The skin may appear inflamed as if burned; however, an actual burn will not occur. OC spray does not cause dermatitis or skin discoloration.[7]

OC spray has come under attack because a number of deaths were seemingly linked to its use. A study conducted by the International Association of Chiefs of Police investigated 30 incidents that occurred between August 1990 and December 1993 in which a person died after being sprayed with OC. The population studied were all males, ranging in age from 24 to 53. In 23 of the 30 incidents, drugs and/or alcohol were found in the bloodstream of the deceased. In the cases where a reasonable conclusion on the cause of death could be determined, OC was not listed as either the cause or a contributor. The study did show that in the majority of cases, death was attributable to "positional asphyxia, aggravated by drugs, disease, and/or obesity." (Positional asphyxia is discussed in Chapter 20.)[8]

Although OC spray itself may be harmless, it can aggravate preexisting medical conditions. For example, in North Carolina, a violent intoxicated person was sprayed with OC and then transported to the local police station where he vomited, aspirated the material, and subsequently died.[9]

If you are requested to provide medical treatment to a suspect who has been sprayed with this substance, first ensure that the suspect has been searched, handcuffed, and properly secured. Because OC spray can cause a localized burning sensation with skin contact, always wear appropriate gloves. If your hands come in contact with the substance, do not touch your face, eat, drink, smoke, or use toilet facilities until you thoroughly wash your hands. Do not let the patient rub the eyes, because this will entrench the cayenne pepper and prolong and intensify the effects. Flush the eyes in accordance with standard procedure; you may also consider removing any contaminated clothing. Some situations may dictate the use of larger volumes of water, using showers or low-pressure hose lines. Law enforcement and fire department/ EMS personnel can use a non-oil base soap to remove the resin, although this is not appropriate in the field. Pat dry the affected area (do not rub) with a cloth towel, taking care not to reuse contaminated portions. It is imperative that patients be properly and continuously monitored to identify any preexisting medical conditions that may be aggravated by the spray. Those conditions would be dealt with according to local standard protocol.

Patients should be transported in a semi-Fowler's position when possible. If the patient continues to exhibit the potential for violence, he or she should be placed in a left laterally recumbent position on a backboard and secured appropriately. All individuals sprayed with an aerosol restraint spray and restrained by any means must be continually monitored during transport. Hospital staff should be made aware of the contamination problem before the patient arrives at the facility.

Light/Sound Diversionary Devices

As with most other products, the light/sound diversionary device or flash bang is manufactured by a number of companies (**Figure 18-4**). These devices have been used by law enforcement and the military since the mid 1970s. These products generate powerful light and sound, producing involuntary reactions by the suspect. The reaction to a 2 million-candle-power flash and a 175-decibel bang leaves most people incapable of any resistance for 6 to 10 seconds. This gives police ample time to enter and secure the area before the suspect can retrieve and use a firearm or other weapon.

Although the flash bang may look like a grenade, it should not be called a "stun grenade." A grenade is a container filled with an explosive compound that causes fragmentation of the container into shrapnel. A flash bang contains no explosive, and the container is not designed to fragment.

Flash bang devices cause few injuries because officers must see where they throw the product. If the fuse device separates from the barrel of the mechanism and is propelled across a room, it can cause injury. In addition, if the device lands next to a small object, the object may be propelled as a secondary missile.

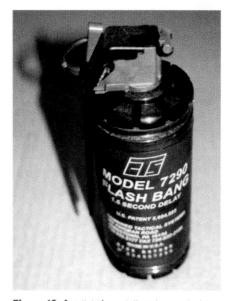

Figure 18-4 A light/sound diversionary device a 2 million-candle-power momentary flash and a 175-decibel bang.

Tasers

The Thomas A. Swift Electronic Rifle (Taser) is another tool police can use to control violent or potentially violent suspects (**Figure 18-5**). This high-voltage, low-energy device is designed to immobilize a suspect temporarily and has been effective in 80% of the incidents where it was deployed (Los Angeles Police Department, Los Angeles, CA, Expanded Course Outline on the Taser TE-93, unpublished material).

The Taser fires two darts attached to fine conducting wires (**Figure 18-6**). Both darts must affix to either the skin or clothing of the suspect for the device to be effective. Once the darts are in place, the officer initiates the 50,000 volt pulsating electrical current for 5 to 10 seconds. New units develop up to 26 watts. The current will pass through 2" of clothing. The electrical energy generated by the device overcomes the body's own electrical system and causes involuntary muscle contractions and loss of motor control. The weapon's effects only last a few minutes.

There are a number of contraindications for using the Taser. Obviously, it should not be used on children, the elderly, or adults weighing less than 80 lb. Taser use should be avoided if the suspect is in a position where he could fall to his death or become entangled in machinery. Use is also contraindicated if the suspect is known to have a history of cardiac disease, a pacemaker, or a neuromuscular disorder such as epilepsy, multiple sclerosis, or muscular dystrophy. Taser users should also check the compatibility of chemical agents that they normally use. If the chemical agent has a flammable component, the addition of 50,000 volts of electricity could be disastrous.

Suspects who have been shot with a Taser should be medically cleared. Darts that hit the skin will generally not penetrate more than ¼" into the skin. Many jurisdictions continue to transport prisoners, with darts imbedded in the skin, to a medical facility for removal. One man-

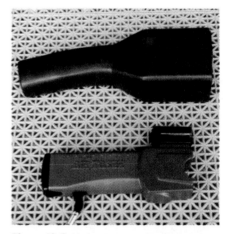

Figure 18-5 Neither version of the Thomas A. Swift Electronic Rifle (TASER) looks like a rifle.

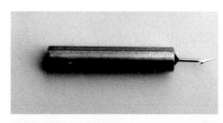

Figure 18-6 Darts fired from a TASER contain barbs similar to a fishhook.

ufacturer notes that if the only medical condition is the darts, either law enforcement or EMS can remove them on the scene (e-mail correspondence with Steve Tuttle, Director of Government and Law Enforcement Affairs, TASER International, April 24, 2001). Agencies should develop response policies and procedures for these incidents.

Projectile Weapons

Less-lethal munitions in the form of projectiles fired from a weapon have been in existence since the 1960s.[10] One of the first was a wooden baton shell developed in the mid 1960s. The device was skip-fired at the legs of rioters in Hong Kong.[11] The rubber bullet was pioneered by the British military and used extensively in Northern Ireland. The original delivery device, a gas grenade launcher, was not very accurate. In 1979, the British army developed the ARWEN (Anti-Riot Weapon, Enfield), a rifle-barrel 37-mm weapon accurate to nearly 100 yards. Today rubber bullet rounds can be delivered by either a 37-mm/40-mm weapon or a 12-gauge shotgun.

Less-lethal projectiles derive their effectiveness from the kinetic energy transferred to the body when the projectile strikes. The pain inflicted and the shock of being hit will, hopefully, incapacitate the suspect long enough for police to take control. Under the formula used by the ballistics industry (kinetic energy = ½ mass × velocity^2), the energy coming from one of these rounds depends heavily on velocity.[2,12] An increase in kinetic energy not only has more potential to incapacitate a person, it also carries a higher risk of producing serious injury or death. Most less-lethal rounds develop velocities from 200 to 325 feet per second. Some rounds, as in the 12-gauge high-velocity rubber pellet round marketed by Defense Technology Corporation of America, have a velocity of 900 feet per second (Defense Technology Corporation of America, Product Specification Manual). But focusing solely on velocity to determine a how lethal a round can be is misleading. A .22-caliber bullet has nearly the same kinetic energy as a bean-bag round launched from a 12-gauge shotgun. The energy from the bullet is concentrated in a very small area, resulting in penetration. The energy from the bean bag is spread over a larger area, causing blunt force trauma (**Figure 18-7 A–C**).

Less-lethal rounds come with a variety of submunitions, the objects that actually leave the barrel of the weapon. These can range from a

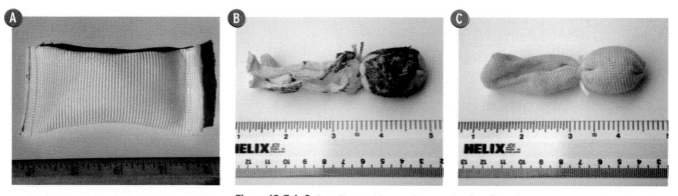

Figure 18-7 A–C Bean bag rounds come in a variety of configurations.

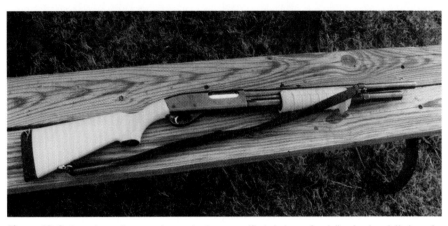

Figure 18-8 Some law enforcement agencies have specified shotguns for delivering less-lethal munitions. In this case the weapon is of a green color to differentiate it from standard 12-gauge shotguns.

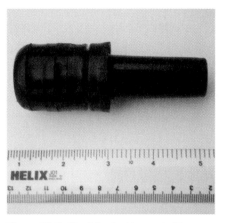

Figure 18-9 Direct-fired rubber projectile.

12-gauge round that fires a single 1.8-cm rubber ball to a 37-mm round that delivers 225 .81-cm rubber balls (**Figure 18-8**). One cartridge delivers three to five wood or rubber batons, while another delivers a single fin-stabilized 5.8-g projectile. Most of these rounds are designed to be direct fired; the weapon is pointed at the suspect and the intent is to have the projectile strike the person directly (**Figure 18-9**). Some of the wooden and rubber baton projectiles are designed to be skip fired (**Figure 18-10 A-B**). The weapon is aimed at the ground in front of a subject and fired so the projectiles strike the ground first and bounce up to the person. The effective range of both the skip-fired and direct-fired rounds varies with manufacturer and type of round. The effective range, according to manufacturer specifications, can be as little as 10' or as much as 190', although most are only effective to about 50'.

Combined Tactical Systems, Inc., markets a StingBall Grenade. As the name implies, this is a grenade that expels a number of small rubber balls in a circular pattern. It also makes a bright flash and a loud bang similar to a sound/light distraction device (**Figure 18-11 A-B**). An irritant powder (CN, CS, or OC) can also be added. As with some distraction devices, the fuse assembly will separate from the body of the grenade.

The objective of less lethal munitions is to incapacitate an individual and limit the ability for further aggressive action. Although these

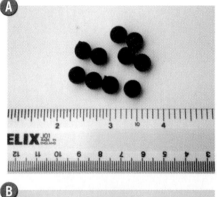
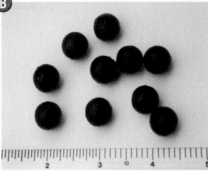

Figure 18-11 A. .31-caliber rubber balls. **B.** .50-caliber rubber balls. Similar size balls are used in 37-mm rounds.

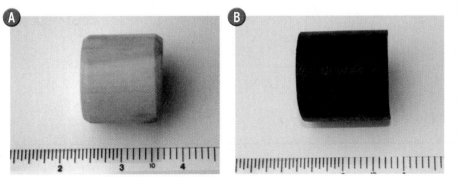

Figure 18-10 A-B Wooden and rubber skip-fired projectiles.

devices are intended to incapacitate rather than kill, serious injuries and deaths do occur. Over the past 20 years, there have been 17 deaths in Northern Ireland from plastic baton rounds.[13] There have been five deaths documented in the past 25 years in the United States and Canada.[14] Of these, two resulted from internal injuries when the projectile fractured ribs; one resulted from a fatal arrhythmia when a bean-bag round stuck the person's sternum; one resulted when the bean-bag round struck the person's throat, and the last resulted when the bean-bag round penetrated the chest and lodged in the heart.

A study of 200 less-lethal munition incidents across the country showed that 53% of the injuries sustained were simple bruising, 20% were abrasions, and only 4.1% involved any penetration of the skin surface.

The primary target areas for less-lethal rounds are the legs, the lower arms, the lower abdomen, and the buttocks. If the suspect has a weapon or if shots to the primary target areas do not produce the desired effect, other areas such as the chest may be targeted. A moving target presents a problem. A round intended to strike the lower abdomen may hit the kidneys if the suspect decides to turn and run.

The possibility of death or serious injury exists whenever a less-lethal round strikes the head, the neck, or the throat and, to a lesser degree, the chest. In an incident involving the use of less-lethal rounds, a thorough examination of the patient is warranted. An impact to the chest may fracture a rib, resulting in pneumothorax or hemothorax. A round that strikes the abdomen may injure a variety of solid or hollow organs. Because the abdominal cavity can hold a large volume of blood, this area deserves close scrutiny.

The use of various less-lethal munitions and chemical agents by law enforcement is increasing. You should realize that these devices or agents may aggravate some preexisting medical conditions. Symptoms may be delayed or masked by drugs or alcohol. Thus, close monitoring is appropriate.

SURVIVAL TIPS

1. Patients exposed to any type of chemical agent should be decontaminated before they are transported.

2. Commercial products are available to neutralize some chemical agents.

3. Do not carry or use any type of chemical agent or less-lethal device unless you are trained in its use and authorized by your agency.

Chapter 19

Civil Disturbances

Many emergency responders have come to accept the violent nature of today's society. Shootings, stabbings, domestic assaults, and drug use are almost routine in some communities. The civil disturbance, however, is one violent situation not routinely faced by most firefighters and emergency medical technicians.

The large scale riots of the 1960s that affected many major cities are one form of civil disturbance. More recently, the Los Angeles riots of April 1992 resulted in the deaths of 53 people and over $1 billion in damage.[1] During the disturbance, the Los Angeles Fire Department responded to over 45,000 fire-related incidents (**Figure 19-1**).[2] Civil disturbances may also be associated with some type of racial discord with-

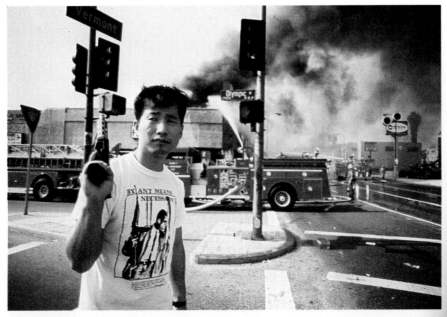

Figure 19-1 During the 1992 Los Angeles riots, 53 people lost their lives. Countless others were injured, including a firefighter.

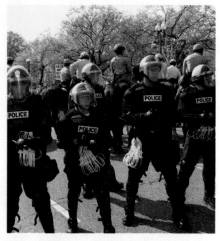

Figure 19-2 Police officers prepare to confront demonstrators at the World Bank meeting in Washington, DC Demonstrations and civil disturbances are by nature very violent events. *(Courtesy Corbis-Sygma)*

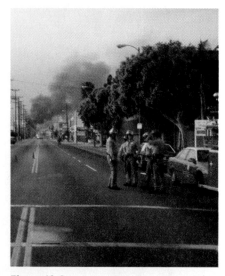

Figure 19-3 Access into the impact area will be limited. The Incident Commander may not be able to obtain normal resources during a civil disturbance. *(Courtesy Captain Patrick Shanley, Los Angeles City Fire Department, CA)*

in a given community. But closer examination shows that civil disturbances occur for a variety of reasons, many of which do not involve racial harmony. Civil disturbances may include the celebrations that result in a devastated downtown area after a city wins a major sports championship, the unrest on a college campus after an unpopular ruling by the Board of Regents, the looting and burning that can accompany a weather event or large scale power outage, and the political demonstrations that center around major international meetings such as the World Trade Organization (**Figure 19-2**). Although these civil disturbances may not match the scale of the Los Angeles riots, they can still tax the ability of local responders to provide adequate, safe service.

Planning

Preparation and planning are key to a safe and efficient operation during a civil disturbance, just as with most other emergencies. Many jurisdictions already have a disaster plan or plans for a major hazardous material incident. But these plans do not address many of the problems that occur during a civil disturbance. Many of the resources that can be called upon to provide assistance during other types of emergencies will not be easily accessible during civil conflict (**Figure 19-3**). For instance, during most major emergencies, getting fuel to equipment is not a major challenge. Fire, EMS, and law enforcement units would have their own fuel units or a private vendor contracted to provide refueling on the incident scene. During a civil disturbance, however, the incident commander must consider what might happen if a vehicle with a substantial load of gasoline or diesel fuel had to pass through an angry crowd armed with Molotov cocktails.

A comprehensive plan must be developed jointly among law enforcement, fire, and EMS services. Any attempt to develop plans for civil unrest without involving associated agencies will ultimately result in failure when a disturbance does erupt. As relationships with local law enforcement develop, police can share intelligence on impending problems with chief officers in fire and rescue services. This advance warning gives chief officers time to review plans and prepare resources for the potential problem.

Based on their experience and knowledge of the circumstances, law enforcement can at times predict when and where a disturbance is probable. For example, a demonstration by a white supremacist group in front of the state legislative building may set the stage for problems. Because such rallies or demonstrations require that the group obtains a permit, authorities can begin planning well in advance. Planning should include a threat assessment conducted jointly by the local fire-and-rescue service and law enforcement. (See Chapter 14 for more information on conducting threat assessments.) The assessment should cover issues such as:

- the anticipated number of protesters
- the possibility of counter-demonstrations
- the history of violence by any involved group
- the ability to contain trouble to a localized geographic area

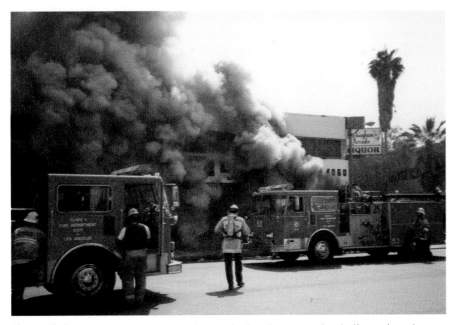

Figure 19-4 The captain, at the cab door, is preparing to put on personal protective equipment over his body armor. *(Courtesy Captain Patrick Shanley, Los Angeles City Fire Department, CA)*

- the use of chemical agents by law enforcement, and the need for decontamination sites
- the need for landing sites for helicopters evacuating the injured
- the need for security at each site

During a civil disturbance, every emergency responder should be outfitted with body armor (**Figure 19-4**). The possibility of a firefighter or emergency medical technician being shot is too great to allow personnel to enter the area unprotected (**Figure 19-5**). Ideally, your department should require you to wear body armor on all potentially violent responses and should have enough bulletproof vests for each crew member on every apparatus. Unfortunately, most departments do not have an adequate supply of vests.

In planning for a disturbance, administrators should identify sources for body armor for rescuers and fire personnel. If a vendor in the area manufactures these garments, the department may make an agreement to obtain sufficient quantities in an emergency. There may be certain limitations with such an agreement, such as availability after hours or on weekends, payment for the use of the garments, and the length of time needed to obtain and distribute them. If chief officers are included in the intelligence loop, the department should have time to gather the needed armor and distribute them to area units. Another alternative might be the local National Guard or Army Reserve unit. They may have ample supplies of military flak vests that can be used. Although flak vests are not tested to National Institute of Justice standards, they are better than wearing nothing at all. Military flak jackets are designed to protect against fragmentation devices such as hand grenades, not bullets. Because the design of both soft body armor and military flak jackets are similar, the flak jacket will stop many small-caliber handgun

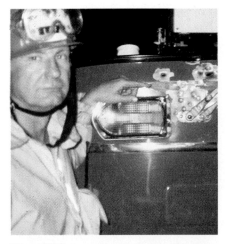

Figure 19-5 Emergency responders will be the target of violence during a civil disturbance. This Los Angeles City Fire Department Captain points to multiple bullet holes from a high-caliber rifle. *(Courtesy Los Angeles City Fire Department, CA)*

rounds. Flak jackets become a viable option when sufficient quantities of soft body armor are not available.

Most departments have procedures for relieving personnel at the scene of a major emergency if the incident extends past the normal rotation of duty shifts. It is not a good idea to allow relief personnel to drive their personal vehicles through the area to the command post or incident scene. This not only endangers the drivers, it also poses an additional problem of vehicle security. Many departments place their personnel on 12-hour shifts; off-duty personnel recuperate at the command post or staging area. Buses with police escort transport rescuers to the incident command post for further deployment.

During the planning stage, base or staging areas should be identified. These locations will serve as command post locations during an incident. Appropriate locations should serve many functions because they will be used as staging areas not only for fire and EMS units but also for police and possibly National Guard units. Schools, stadiums, and military armories are sites that should be considered. During the 1992 disturbance, the Los Angeles Fire Department utilized a bus yard as a command center. With its high block walls, the yard provided some security from rocks and bottles.

The command center serves a variety of needs. As a remote dispatching center, the facility should have sufficient office space with ample phones. As a rehabilitation center, the area should have kitchen facilities, as well as rest rooms and showers. Because personnel may be on a 12-hour rotation, consideration should be given to dormitory facilities. Most disaster plans should have already identified sources for large quantities of cots. If it is normal practice during disasters to have inmates from local prisons prepare and serve food, would such a practice be appropriate during a civil disturbance? If apparatus is normally staffed with two or three people, increasing staff to a minimum of four people is warranted.

Most departments will not be able to handle a disturbance of any magnitude without mutual aid from neighboring jurisdictions. If these areas are also experiencing unrest, the situation becomes even more complicated. The call for mutual aid may go to the far reaches of the state and may even cross state boundaries. When any mutual aid companies respond to such an incident, a variety of problems can arise. Some of these issues, such as common radio frequencies or the need for area maps, may be identified during a mutual aid response for routine emergencies and should be resolved through normal disaster planning.

If mutual aid assistance is requested, consideration should be given to requesting strike teams or task forces. One decision facing the chief officer who sends his units to another jurisdiction during a civil disturbance is that of security. Should he send his personnel with the hope that adequate police units will be assigned to protect them or does he have police from his jurisdiction respond with the team to ensure adequate security? Such a decision must be made in the planning stage because a variety of legal and legislative issues must be addressed. Unless specifically noted, police from one jurisdiction may not have police powers in another even during a crisis.

Many departments have written documents containing their plans for major disasters, hazardous materials incidents, and even day-to-day operations. Given the unique circumstances of a civil disturbance, plans for such an event should also be written and kept available for reference. Once a year the plans should be taken out, reviewed, and revised where needed.

Strategy

Once a disturbance has erupted, task-force or strike-team operations should be implemented as quickly as possible. If warning of such an event has been provided, task forces may be readied in anticipation of problems. Task forces are generally three-engine companies, one ladder company, and a command level officer. A strike team is five engine companies with a command level officer. Either a task force or a strike team will respond to each reported incident. For safety, the task force or strike team will move as a cohesive unit. Allowing one unit to respond alone is dangerous and should be avoided. In addition, each task force or strike team should have a law enforcement or military escort (**Figure 19-6**). Preferably, there should be at least four police officers or military personnel assigned as escorts to each task force. One of the officers or soldiers should ride with the command officer. At no time should a team respond with fewer than two escort personnel. Each firefighter or paramedic should be issued body armor before entering the impact area. Note: Fire and EMS personnel should never carry firearms unless specifically sanctioned by their agency (tactical medics, or arson investigators).

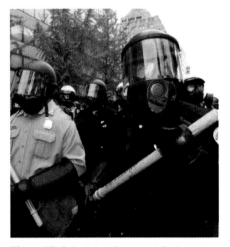

Figure 19-6 Each task force or strike team should have ample police security assigned. *(Courtesy Corbis-Sygma)*

The strategy used during a civil disturbance is unlike any other operation. Most departments have adequate resources to handle routine emergencies in their district. On large incidents, additional manpower and apparatus can be requested with the expectation that it will arrive within a reasonable time frame. During a civil disturbance, resources are at a premium. An incident that would normally be handled by two to three alarms of equipment might be the responsibility of a single task force (**Figure 19-7**). Additional apparatus may quite simply not be avail-

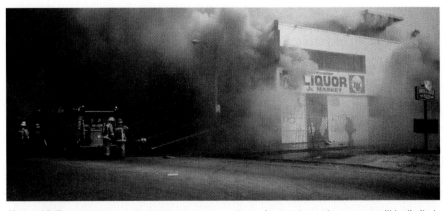

Figure 19-7 Incidents normally handled by large numbers of apparatus and manpower will be limited during a civil disturbance. *(Courtesy Captain Patrick Shanley, Los Angeles City Fire Department, CA)*

able. If there is a high call volume, department officials may be forced to respond to structure fires only. This means that dumpsters, cars, and other items will be allowed to burn unless they threaten a structure.

Task force commanders should also consider their own team's limitations. Initiating operations on a fully involved 200' × 200' commercial building may not be the wisest strategy if there is a second structure down the street that has smoke showing from the first floor. If resources are limited, the most appropriate decision may be to bypass the fully involved building and focus on the structure that can be saved.

Operational strategies on the scene will also be quite different from routine strategies. During a civil disturbance, engine companies should quickly knock down the fire and move on to the next incident. Large caliber streams from deluge sets and 2½" hand lines should be employed. Rooftop operations should be limited to those incidents where a hazard to life exists. If call volume is heavy, units should also avoid time-consuming salvage and overhaul operations. The only salvage operation that might be considered is to place a building's sprinkler system back in service because this may save the structure from future arson attempts.

Tactics

If the potential for a disturbance is identified through early intelligence gathering and planning, there are a number of deployment activities that companies may use not only to increase efficiency but also to reduce the potential of injury to personnel. For example, if possible, use only those units with fully enclosed cabs. Examine your vehicles and apparatus. Are there tools such as ceiling hooks, pry bars, axes, or halogen tools mounted on the exterior that someone could grab and use as a weapon against the crew? If so, place them in compartments. Remove nonessential items like salvage covers, submersible pumps, and fans that will not be used. Replace these items with extra drinking water, clothing items for crew members, and food. Civil disturbances may last hours, days, or weeks, and provide little opportunity for a crew to return to quarters. Even though interior attack is only recommended where a life hazard exists, the resupply of air bottles for self-contained breathing apparatus (SCBA) may be limited. If additional air bottles are kept at the station, they should be moved to a place on the apparatus.

If the station is being used as a staging area for apparatus entering the impact area, a floor watch or guard should be maintained at all times. Window shades should be drawn so that personnel within the building are not easy targets for any would-be gunmen. If the station is being vacated or abandoned, electrical power to the fueling pumps should be shut down. This reduces the possibility that someone will steal gasoline or diesel fuel to make firebombs. Remove the radio microphone from the station radio so that intruders cannot tie-up radio frequencies. Take any reserve equipment housed in the station to the staging area. It could be used later for additional crews or to replace a disabled unit. Secure personal automobiles belonging to the crew in the empty apparatus bays to reduce the possibility of returning to a damaged or stolen vehicle.

Once task forces are established, team commanders should brief their personnel, including law enforcement or military personnel assigned to

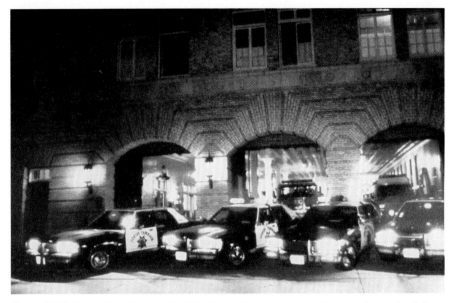

Figure 19-8 Cooperative efforts put forth by fire and law enforcement will ensure the safety of all personnel. *(Courtesy Los Angeles City Fire Department, CA)*

the task force (**Figure 19-8**). The briefing should include information on safety issues and operational tactics. The task force commander should ensure that all agencies know which radio frequencies will be used, what the agreed-upon emergency code words or signals are, and what tactics will be used if an emergency extraction is necessary. Signals might include one long airhorn blast by all on-scene equipment to initiate an evacuation/extraction.

All personnel should be reminded of the need for task force integrity. No one unit should leave the task force for any reason. Once on-scene, personnel should maintain the buddy system and remain in groups of no fewer than two people. The briefing should also include a quick review of the strategies and tactics that will be employed by firefighters. Law enforcement and military personnel will also find this information helpful in planning the interactions needed to provide adequate security. Any suggestions by law enforcement that may bolster security should also be included in the briefing.

At the incident scene, the task force commander and his police counterpart should conduct an initial size-up. The size-up should include a few additional items not considered during routine operations. For example, is there a crowd near the area? How many people are there? Do they appear hostile? Are the police escorts confident in their ability to secure this scene? Are there multi-story buildings nearby where snipers might be waiting? Are there helicopters available to assess the surrounding area? Is the fire so large that the structure cannot be saved?

The preferred strategy during a civil disturbance is to extinguish structure fires as quickly as possible with little or no salvage and overhaul. Engine companies should use deluge streams and handlines wherever practical (**Figure 19-9**). This provides quick knock-down and hastens the company's return to service for assignment to another incident. Vertical ventilation from rooftops should be avoided because firefighters on these remote positions become easy targets. A circle-the-wagons

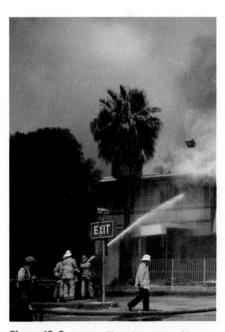

Figure 19-9 Large-caliber streams provide quick knock-down when hit-and-run tactics are employed. *(Courtesy Captain Patrick Shanley, Los Angeles City Fire Department, CA)*

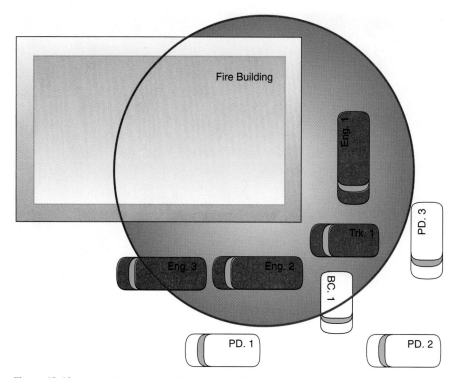

Figure 19-10 Appropriate placement of apparatus at incident scene.

approach should be used, with units placed around the building with pump panels facing the structure (**Figure 19-10**). This provides cover and concealment for both firefighters and pump operators. Units should not be isolated from one another. Placing one company on each side of the structure, for instance, may be the best use of limited resources but may not be the best option for scene security.

Fire units should also be aware that a quick retreat may be necessary at any time. For this reason, the use of master stream devices from aerial ladders should be limited because retracting and bedding the aerial ladder and disconnecting any hoselines takes time. If the company must retreat, there may be insufficient time to disconnect and repack the hoselines. If violence erupts, it may be appropriate to drive quickly away from a hydrant, even if doing so results in a broken hose connection. If possible, small alleys and dead-end streets should be avoided because it is difficult to retreat from those areas.

Many local and state law enforcement agencies maintain helicopters for aerial reconnaissance. Fire department officials should use this resource whenever possible during a civil disturbance. Placing a command-level officer high above a disturbance has several advantages. The airborne officer can provide a responding task force with an alternate route of travel around an angry mob and will be able to observe the extent of the fire problem. Are there 5 or 25 structures burning?

EMS Unit Tactics

EMS units should also be configured in task forces consisting of at least one engine company, advanced life support or paramedic capability if available, and two transport units. The level of care that can be provided will be dictated by the available resources. Each medical task force should have at least 4 police officers or military personnel assigned to provide escort security. At least 1 EMS task force should be kept in reserve for care and transport of injured police officers and firefighters. Providing adequate care for rescuers should be of primary concern.

With few exceptions, the EMS system response to civil disturbances is the same as for other disasters. Casualty collection points and remote treatment areas should be established if necessary. This will reduce the load on hospitals by enabling treatment of minor injuries in the field. If space allows, command post and staging areas may also be appropriate sites for the collection points, thus reducing the number of personnel required for security at a separate facility. However, the operation of a command post or staging facility must not be hindered by the operations at a casualty collection point just as the operation of the casualty collection point should not be hampered by other operations. If problems are anticipated, another area or facility should be used. If appropriate, a section of the collection point may be set up as a temporary morgue. Check local disaster plans for specifics on establishing both temporary morgues, casualty collection points, or remote treatment areas.

Treatment of casualties in an exposed area during a civil disturbance should be limited. Patients should be quickly moved to the ambulance for transport. This reduces the exposure of personnel to possible violence from crowds or hidden snipers. The patient can be treated while en route to a casualty collection point or other treatment facility. Jurisdictions should also consider whether a no-code policy would be appropriate during a disturbance. This policy considers all patients without a pulse or respirations as expired. Attempts to revive a cardiac arrest patient within an impact area leave personnel exposed and hold limited resources on one incident for an extended period of time.

SURVIVAL TIPS

1. During a civil disturbance, personnel should remove collar ornaments, badges, name plates, and all extraneous materials from their uniforms.

2. A person on a ladder is an easy target for gunmen. No one should be exposed to this risk.

3. Any food or drink offered by citizens to rescuers should be graciously refused; they could be poisoned.

4. Duct tape in the shape of the letter X should be placed on the side windows of all apparatus. If a window is struck by a hard object, the glass will not shatter into the faces of crew members.

5. To ensure safety, all crew members should wear all bunker gear while enroute to or returning from incidents during a civil disturbance.

Chapter# Chapter 20

Patient Restraint

One of the most troubling decisions faced by emergency responders is when and how to restrain a patient. In these cases, both action and inaction can result in death of the patient and legal liability for both you and your agency (**Figure 20-1**). The problem of restraint also plagues the law enforcement community. In 1994, a number of in-custody deaths originally thought to be linked to the use of pepper spray were later attributed to what is now identified as positional asphyxia.[1]

The typical positional asphyxia scenario involves an individual taken into custody by the police. This person engages in a physical confrontation with officers, during which pulse and respirations increase. Perhaps this person has recently ingested a moderate quantity of alcohol. The

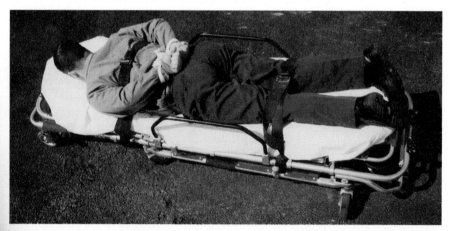

Figure 20-1 Emergency responders have been taught a number of techniques to restrain patients. Some can cause injury or death, such as this one. *Never* restrain a patient in this position.

officers, following standard procedure, handcuff the individual, hands behind his back. If the confrontation continues, officers use a leash-type device to wrap the ankles. The leash is then attached to the handcuffs and the feet are drawn back and up toward the hands, a procedure known as hog-tying. The suspect is then placed in the rear of a police vehicle in a prone, or face-down, position. By the time the suspect arrives at the police station, he is no longer breathing.

Donald Reay, MD, a medical examiner in King County, Washington, examined many in-custody deaths and testified at the subsequent court cases involving these deaths. According to Dr. Reay, several factors may contribute to positional asphyxia. The individuals involved were drug and/or alcohol intoxicated, possibly mentally unstable, and in a violent struggle with law enforcement. In addition, each had a large abdomen, which could contribute to the development of hypoxia.

Dr. Reay concluded that placing individuals with large abdomens in the prone position forces the abdominal contents up against the diaphragm. This would limit movement of the diaphragm in breathing. Because the diaphragm is critical to respiratory function, this limitation would eventually lead to decreased blood oxygen levels, hypoxia, cardiac dysrhythmias, and death.

EMS Court Cases

A number of similar incidents have also occurred during prehospital care. Patients who were restrained face-down on a stretcher have died despite the presence of advanced life support providers.

One such incident occurred in February 1991. Initial attempts to secure the patient, who was experiencing seizures and was very combative, were unsuccessful. Paramedics and firefighters finally secured the man face-down, using a ladder strap to hold his wrists and ankles. Before the patient arrived at the hospital, he stopped breathing. Resuscitative efforts were initiated immediately and continued at the hospital emergency department, but the patient died 7 days later. Both the jurisdiction and its fire department were sued for gross negligence, and the case was settled for over $330,000.[2]

In another incident, police secured a combative, agitated man with handcuffs and hobble restraints. Paramedics were apparently summoned in response to the man's mental state. The patient was attached to a cardiac monitor and placed in a prone position on the stretcher. Paramedics watched as the patient's heart rhythm became unstable and finally went into cardiac arrest. Despite immediate resuscitative efforts, the patient died. The autopsy noted that both amphetamine and methamphetamine were present in his blood stream.[3]

In December 1993, an EMS unit responded to transport an individual in police custody. The man had possible injuries resulting from the arrest. When they arrived, emergency responders found the subject still combative. They placed the patient prone on a stretcher and covered him with a full-body-length canvas tarp with straps on each corner, similar to the sandwiching technique noted in many prehospital care textbooks. The patient's position and the handcuffs made taking a pulse difficult, but a capillary refill test was completed. Upon arrival at the hospital, the man was in cardiac arrest, and attempts to resuscitate him were unsuccessful. The decedent's family filed suit claiming gross negligence. Specifically noted in the plaintiff's case was the responders' use of the canvas restraining device. Although the case was dismissed by the United States Court of Appeals, the emergency responders were kept on an emotional seesaw with court appearances, depositions, and affidavits until the decision was final—in August 1997, nearly 4 years later.[4]

Criteria for Restraint

Emergency responders must recognize that a person may become aggressive and combative for many reasons, including psychological disorders, drugs, alcohol, trauma to certain body systems, and some metabolic disorders like hypoglycemia. However, some people are just simply mean and nasty.

Fire and rescue services should develop policies governing the application of restraints. Generally, restraints should only be used if these criteria are met:

- The patient is a danger to himself or herself (suicidal, attempting to remove IVs).
- There is an underlying medical or trauma condition that is causing the combativeness (head injury, hypoglycemia).
- The person is a danger to others, including the responders attempting to help (alcohol, drugs, behavior).
- The person is in police custody and must be transported to a medical facility for treatment of a medical or trauma-related problem.

If any one of these criteria is met, physical restraint may be indicated. If a patient must be physically restrained, law enforcement should be summoned.

Restraint Procedures

Many jails and prisons have developed restraint teams. These specially trained guards follow specific policies and procedures to reduce the possibility of injury to both the combative inmate and the guards themselves. Members of these teams routinely train with the procedures. When called upon, these groups develop a plan of action and each member is given a specific assignment. Emergency responders may not be able to call upon specialized teams, but can learn from the techniques used by such teams. Fire and EMS departments should not only have policies in place to determine the need for restraint, they should also have procedures describing how the person should be restrained.

If a patient must be physically restrained, the highest ranking member or officer-in-charge (OIC) of the emergency crew should, if time permits, develop a plan of action. Obviously, any plan should be discussed with police before it is implemented. The OIC should have specific assignments for each member of the restraint team. For example, one crew member might be assigned to control the left arm, another crew member assigned to the right leg and a third crew member to the head. Such a detailed plan will not always be possible. A quickly changing situation may require action with limited resources and planning.

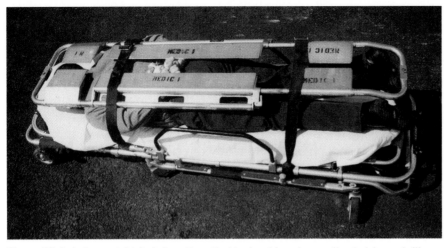

Figure 20-2 In the sandwich technique, the patient is placed face-down on the stretcher and either a backboard or scoop-stretcher is placed over the patient. This technique should **never** be used.

A person being restrained must **never** be placed face-down (**Figure 20-2**). The patient should be placed supine or in a left laterally recumbent position. This will significantly reduce the possibility of positional asphyxia. Using a typical backboard and straps may be an effective restraint. Because spinal stabilization is both common and medically acceptable, responders should consider it as the primary means of restraint (**Figure 20-3**).

Any restraining devices such as leather restraints must be medically acceptable. Homemade restraint devices must not be used or carried in an emergency response unit. If a patient being restrained by such a device dies, both the responder and the department may face civil litigation.

Recent Developments

A recent California incident has further confused the issue of patient restraint and positional asphyxia. In 1994, a 35-year-old San Diego man was hog-tied and later died in custody. The medical examiner stated

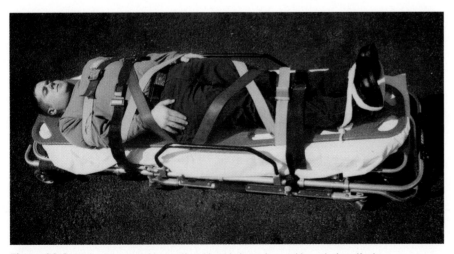

Figure 20-3 Medically acceptable practices should always be used to restrain patients.

that the cause of death was "restrictive asphyxia" resulting from "maximum restraint in a prone position by law enforcement."[5] The man's family filed a wrongful death suit against San Diego County. The University of California at San Diego (UCSD) Medical Center was called upon to conduct a study on hog-tying and positional asphyxia. The study, conducted by Thomas Neuman, MD, found that although the position may limit a person's ability to breathe it does not affect blood oxygen and carbon dioxide levels. Any mechanical impairment was so minor that it would not cause asphyxia.[6] This study directly contradicted the theory proposed by Dr. Reay as described earlier. In court, Dr. Reay retracted his own findings after learning about the UCSD study. The judge in the case noted, "Like a house of cards, the evidence for positional asphyxia has fallen completely," and later dismissed the case.[7]

Both Drs. Reay and Neuman agree that further study is needed. Until conclusive evidence is available, emergency responders should avoid placing combative patients in a prone position.

Documentation

Whenever a patient must be restrained, it is critical that the actions of emergency medical personnel be well documented. Note what criteria was used to determine the need for restraint and what specific actions were taken during the restraint procedure. The crew should also note all patient monitoring during transport, including pulse, blood pressure, respiration, skin color and temperature, and neurologic status.

SURVIVAL TIPS

1) Never restrain a patient in a prone position.

2) Frequently monitor the vital signs of patients in restraints.

Chapter 21

Terrorism: Calibrating Risks and Response*

Terrorist events are not new to our world. Recent events clearly delineate the devastation that these acts can and do yield. Consider, for example, the bombings of the New York City World Trade Center (1993 and 2001), the Murrah Federal Building in Oklahoma City (**Figure 21-1 A-B**), Khobar Towers in Saudi Arabia, the United States embassies in Kenya and Tanzania, and the USS Cole; the nerve gas attack by Aum Shinrikyo in the Tokyo subway; and the arrest of three members of the militia group "Republic of Texas" in their plot to kill former President Clinton and key federal officials using an improvised biologic weapons delivery system that involved modified BIC lighters rigged to inject anthrax, HIV, and rabies through the skin via a coated cactus thorn.[1]

These incidents, along with others that law enforcement agencies have interdicted, illustrate, with increasing and alarming frequency, how

*Author: Paul M. Maniscalco MPA, PhD(c), EMT-P. Deputy Chief with New York City Fire Department. Adj. Asst. Professor, The George Washington University. Member, Gilmore National Terrorism Commission

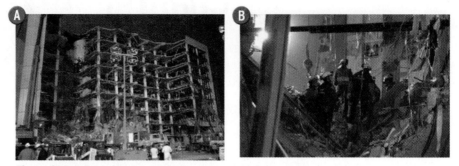

Figure 21-1 A-B The bombing of the Murrah Federal Building in Oklahoma City shows that any community is vulnerable to a terrorist act. (*Courtesy Paul M. Maniscalco*)

terrorism has become a complex issue confronting state and local emergency response organizations.

Overview

There are many different definitions of terrorism. For the purposes of this chapter, the following definition is used:

Terrorism is the use of violence, threats, intimidation, or information manipulation for revenge, politics, support of a cause or the furthering of a criminal enterprise.[2]

Terrorist incidents take various forms, most commonly involving explosives.[3] Recently, other methods have gotten more attention because of the greater threat and level of risk associated with them (**Figure 21-2**). These weapons or potential attack forms are addressed by the United States' domestic policy on counter-terrorism.

The phrase "weapons of mass destruction" (WMD) emerged as the buzzword for terrorism in the late 1990s. The term attempts to convey the significant consequences of these devices or substances. In this chapter, however, the phrase "weapons of mass effect" (WME) will be used because using these weapons will not assure literal destruction but will realize various degrees of effects. These weapon types are:

- Biologics and biologic weapons: the use of biologic substances (etiologic agents) as weapons or the use of delivery systems (weaponization) for biologic distribution in an attack

- Chemicals and chemical weapons: the use of chemicals as weapons or the use of delivery systems (weaponization) for chemical distribution in an attack

- Cyberterrorism: the use of rogue computer commands (viruses) or unauthorized entry into computerized systems to damage, render useless, or promulgate incorrect or inaccurate data operations

- High explosives: the use of military grade explosives

- Radiologic or nuclear terrorism: the use of radiologic material or the use of weaponized nuclear material to cause damage

The major issue for local emergency responders is coordinating with law enforcement agencies to identify the existing threat while also calibrating the risk so that an effective response plan can be developed.

Recently, many government agencies and institutions have attempted to address the problem of terrorism. In fact, the United States govern-

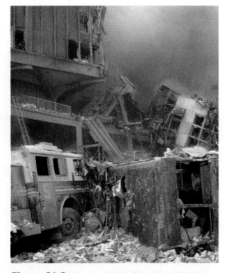

Figure 21-2 The bombing of the World Trade Center in New York City confirmed that explosives are still the choice for many terrorists. (*© Steve Spak/911 Pictures*)

ment has spent almost $10 billion with over 40 different agencies to implement its domestic policy on terrorism and to build a better mouse trap to assist on the front lines.[4] Within a week of the September 11, 2001 attacks, Congress, at the request of the White House, released another $40 billion as an initial emergency fiscal disbursement to cover issues ranging from training and readiness to recovery. Recent events and threat assessments by agencies such as the Department of Defense (**Figure 21-3**), the State Department, the Defense Intelligence Agency, the Central Intelligence Agency, the Secret Service, the Bureau of Alcohol, Tobacco, and Firearms, and the Federal Bureau of Investigation have underscored the importance of understanding the underlying risks and direct ramifications of an attack. In fact, Senator Sam Nunn (D-ret) of Georgia has been frequently quoted as stating, "It is not a question of if…but when…" an incident would occur.[5] Unfortunately for the world, he was proven correct on September 11, 2001.

On a personal note, I am compelled to state that if the emergency response community is expected to be the "first on the scene," then it is not unreasonable to expect that it should be the first to be trained and its organizations the first to be funded to confront this emerging threat[6] (**Figure 21-4**). Clearly this matter needs to be addressed quickly so that the emergency response community can meet its mandate of saving lives and property without losing the lives of its members in a WME terrorist event. I believe that the public safety triad (police, fire, and EMS) are indisputably America's first line of defense in the war against terrorism.

Although no textbook chapter (within the context of page limitations) can provide a full resolution to this matter, this chapter contains an overview of the various types of threats that exist. This synopsis is intended to be thought-provoking and to provide an understanding that these incidents will require a new method of responding to events, different equipment to keep emergency responders safe, dynamic defensive operation strategies that can be adjusted as the threat changes, and a big picture view in composing emergency response plans. When an attack does occur, we know that it will require a statewide, regional, or national response to manage the consequences effectively. Incorporating surrounding communities and counties as well as emergency management personnel in the planning process is greatly encouraged.

Biologic and Chemical Terrorism

Examples of the use of chemicals as weapons can be traced as far back as 423 B.C. when "Spartan allies in the Peloponnesian War took an Athenian-held fort by directing smoke from lighted coals, sulfur, and pitch through a hollowed-out beam into the fort."[7] One only needs to read the local newspapers to witness the frequency and impact of chemical weapon attacks. Recently, chemicals such as butyric acid, a noxious chemical that smells like vomit, have been used as weapons at abortion and family planning clinics. Similar instances of chemical use against clinics have been reported in Dallas, Texas; New Orleans, Louisiana; and several cities in Florida.[8] Although simplistic in execution, these events pose two critical issues for responders, namely, their personal

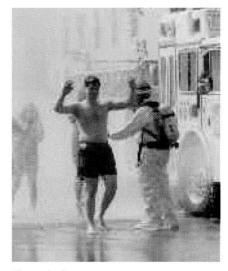

Figure 21-3 A target for terrorist activity: Department of Defense officials conduct an exercise at the Pentagon. *(Courtesy Paul M. Maniscalco)*

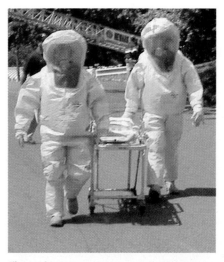

Figure 21-4 Emergency responders from fire, rescue, and law enforcement will be the front line of response to a terrorist attack. *(Courtesy Paul M. Maniscalco)*

safety and the complexities of treating these patients. Clearly, this multi-dimensional problem mandates that local emergency response systems have a sustainable, coordinated, and effective response to hostile emergency scenes.

Chemical Weapons

Chemical weapons are chemical substances that are used on the military battlefield to injure, incapacitate, or kill the adversary. In modern times, the deliberate use of chemicals during World War I and the devastation that resulted were so repugnant that international treaties forbidding the use and manufacture of such weapons were implemented. But in 1995, the unthinkable happened again, when chemical weapons were used on a civilian population in Tokyo, Japan.

At approximately 8:10 AM on March 20, 1995, reports of a toxic fume problem at Tokyo's Hibiya subway line were received. When responders arrived, they found passengers unconscious, vomiting, and seizing. The official report of the number of injuries associated with this event was over 4,500 patients and 12 dead. Of those injured, 700 had extended hospitalizations, including 75 who were categorized in critical condition. The world had witnessed the use of a chemical (sarin) as a weapon on a civilian population by a religious cult known as the Aum Shinrikyo.[2]

As alarming as this organization's use of a chemical as a weapon is, the fact remains that this was only the most successful of a series of attacks or releases that the Aums were responsible for executing over a 3-year period. Below is a brief synopsis of these events:

1. March 15, 1995: Three attaché cases were discovered at a Tokyo subway station. Each case contained three tanks of an unknown liquid, a small motorized fan, a vent, and a battery. One of the cases was giving off a vapor. There has been no confirmation by the Japanese government on what product was used.

2. March 5, 1995: Nineteen people were taken to a hospital after they inhaled fumes in a train car in Yokohama, a port city near Tokyo. Patient complaints centered on eye and respiratory pain. The source of the fumes was not found.

3. January 4, 1995: Aum Shinrikyo filed a complaint accusing a company president of spreading sarin into its religious facilities in Kamikuishiki, a town in central Japan. The company president brought counter charges in February. Reports have linked this cult to several unresolved kidnappings, including the kidnappings of some high profile individuals.

4. December, 1994: Material believed to be sarin was discovered in Kamikuishiki. The investigation is still open.

5. September 1, 1994: More than 231 people in seven towns in the Japanese state of Nara suffered rashes, eye irritation, and respiratory distress from unknown fumes.

6. July 1994: Several residents of Kamikuishiki complained of eye and nose irritation, respiratory difficulty, and nausea resulting from an unknown fume source.

7. June 21, 1994: Seven people died and more than 200 were affect-ed by sarin fumes from an unknown source that spread through a quiet residential area in Matsumoto in central Japan.

8. July 2, 1993: More than 100 residents in Tokyo's Koto district complained about noxious white fumes rising from buildings owned by the Aum cult. City officials were denied entry to the buildings to investigate and no follow-up took place.

The last and most unfortunate Tokyo event has heightened the inter-est of both responders and rogue organizations to the use and impact of chemicals as weapons.

There are many hazardous materials in the world; just take a look at the United States Department of Transportation *2000 North American Emergency Response Guide*. The widespread availability of chemicals that are easily accessed and effective for mass use makes WME even more appealing to a rogue group. Additionally, instructions for constructing chemical weapons and delivery devices are widely available in books and on the World Wide Web.

Intentional releases of hazardous materials as part of a criminal or terrorist act pose unique challenges to responders. This is not a garden-variety HazMat job. Even responders who are trained to traditional haz-ardous materials competencies may encounter unique exposure risks, emergency control challenges, unusual materials, and complex mass casualty situations that are beyond their experiences and control[9] (**Figure 21-5**).

Responders must remain cognizant of two major issues. (1) An industrial chemical or hazardous material can inflict effective and wide-spread damage equivalent to a military agent. (2) Terrorist groups or organizations do not comply with existing HazMat requirements, so the

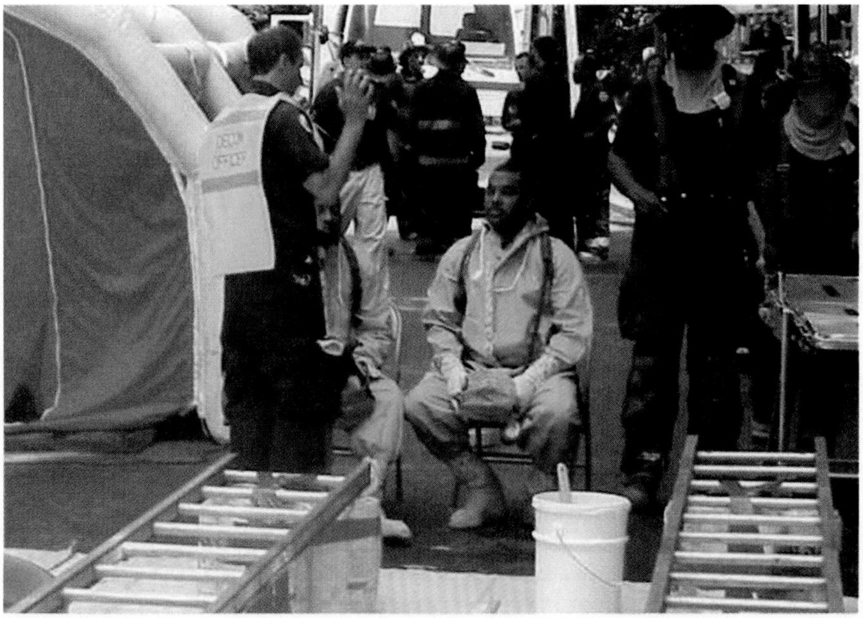

Figure 21-5 A chemical weapons attack can overwhelm even the most well-equipped HazMat teams. *(Courtesy Paul M. Maniscalco)*

event will not have MSDS, UN numbers, or NFPA 401 placards. In most cases, the clinical presentation of the patients will be the biggest clue to the type of substance used. Responders should also remember, as with any hazardous material response, personal safety comes first. Evacuate the area, isolate those affected, and deny entry to nonessential personnel to minimize the patient load.

Military Chemical Agents

Chemical agents used by the military are broken down into five subcategories that reflect their actions on a victim. The five categories are: (1) nerve agents such as tabun (GA), sarin (GB), soman (GD), and V-agent (VX); (2) vesicants or blister agents such as mustard (H), distilled mustard (HD), nitrogen mustard (HN), and lewisite (L); (3) blood agents or cyanides such as hydrogen cyanide (AC) or cyanogen chloride (CK); (4) choking or pulmonary agents such as chlorine (CL) or phosgene (CG); and (5) irritants or riot control agents such as mace and pepper sprays (CS, CR, CN, OC).

Each of these subcategories is classified under the requirements set forth in the *1996 North American Emergency Response Guide* as Class 6.1—toxic/poisonous materials and infectious substances hazardous materials.[10] A general description of each follows and **Table 21-1** summarizes signs and symptoms, decontamination techniques, and treatment steps.

Table 21-1 Chemical Agents

NERVE AGENTS (GA, GB, GD, GF, VX)	MUSTARD (H, HD, HN) *Vesicant/Blister Agents*
Signs and Symptoms: Vapor: *Small exposure*–Miosis, rhinorrhea, and mild dyspnea. *Large exposure*–Sudden loss of consciousness, convulsions, apnea, flaccid paralysis, copious secretions, and miosis. Liquid on skin: *Small to moderate exposure*–Localized sweating, nausea, vomiting, and feeling of weakness. *Large exposure*–Sudden loss of consciousness, convulsions, apnea, flaccid paralysis, and copious secretions.	Unique Characteristic: Sulfur mustard can smell like garlic and/or horseradish. Signs and Symptoms: Asymptomatic latent period (hours). Erythema and blisters on the skin; irritation, conjunctivitis, corneal opacity, and damage in the eyes; mild upper respiratory signs; marked airway damage; also gastrointestinal effects and bone marrow stem cell suppression.
Decontamination: Large amounts of water with a hypochlorite solution.	Decontamination: Large amounts of water with a hypochlorite solution.
Immediate Treatment/Management: Administration of atropine and pralidoxime chloride (2PAM); diazepam if casualty is severe; ventilation and suction of airway for respiratory distress.	Immediate Treatment/Management: Decontamination immediately after exposure is the only way to prevent or limit injury and damage. Symptomatic management of lesions.
LEWISITE (L) *Vesicant/Blister Agent*	**PHOSGENE OXIME (CX)** *Choking Agent*
Unique Characteristic: Can smell like geraniums.	Unique Characteristic: Can smell like fresh-mown hay.

(Continued)

Table 21-1 Chemical Agents *(Continued)*

LEWISITE (L) *Vesicant/Blister Agent*

Signs and Symptoms: Lewisite causes immediate pain or irritation of skin and mucous membranes. Erythema and blisters on the skin and eyes with airway damage similar to that seen after mustard exposure develop later.

Decontamination: Large amounts of water with a hypochlorite solution.

Immediate Treatment/Management: Immediate decontamination; symptomatic management of lesions (the same as for mustard lesions). A specific antidote, British Anti-Lewisite (BAL), will decrease systemic effects.

PHOSGENE OXIME (CX) *Choking Agent*

Signs and Symptoms: Immediate burning and irritation followed by wheal-like skin lesions and eye and airway damage.

Decontamination: Large amounts of water.

Immediate Treatment/Management: Termination of exposure; ABCs of resuscitation; immediate decontamination; enforced rest and observation; oxygen, with or without positive airway pressure, for signs of respiratory distress; symptomatic management of lesions; other supportive therapy as needed.

CYANIDE (AC, CK) *Blood Agents*

Unique Characteristic: Can smell like bitter almonds

Signs and Symptoms: Few; seizures, respiratory and cardiac arrest after exposure to high estimated dose (Ct).

Decontamination: Skin decontamination is usually not necessary because agents are highly volatile. Wet, contaminated clothing should be removed and the underlying skin decontaminated with water or other standard decontaminates.

Treatment: *Antidote:* intravenous sodium nitrite and sodium thiosulfate. *Supportive care:* oxygen and correct acidosis.

PULMONARY AGENTS (CG) *Choking Agents*

Signs and Symptoms: Eye and airway irritation; dyspnea; chest tightness; delayed pulmonary edema.

Decontamination: *Vapor:* fresh air. *Liquid:* copious water irrigation.

Treatment: Termination of exposure; ABCs of resuscitation; enforced rest and observation; oxygen, with or without positive airway pressure, for signs of respiratory distress; other supportive therapy as needed.

RIOT CONTROL AGENTS (CS, CN) *Irritants*

Signs and Symptoms: Burning and pain on exposed mucous membranes and skin; eye pain and tearing; burning nostrils; respiratory discomfort; tingling of the exposed skin.

Decontamination: Thoroughly flush eyes with water, saline, or similar substance. Flush skin with copious amounts of water, alkaline soap and water, or a mildly alkaline solution (sodium bicarbonate or sodium carbonate). Generally decontamination is not required if wind is brisk.

Treatment: Usually none is necessary; effects are self-limiting.

CHLORINGE (CL) *Choking Agents*

Signs and Symptoms: Burning sensation in the upper airways and lungs with an onset of spasmodic coughing, dyspnea and increasing choking; hoarseness or aphonia, followed by stridor; retching and vomiting (gastric contents will smell like chlorine); probable pulmonary edema. *Significant exposures*–rapid onset pulmonary edema with death.

Decontamination: Thoroughly flush eyes with water, saline, or similar substance. Flush skin with copious amounts of water.

Treatment: Termination of exposure; ABCs of resuscitation; enforced rest and observation; oxygen, with or without positive airway pressure, for signs of respiratory distress; other supportive therapy as needed.

Sources: United States Army Medical Research Institute of Chemical Defense: *Medical Management of Chemical Casualties Handbook*, ed 2. Aberdeen Proving Ground, MD, Chemical Casualty Care Office, 1995.

Office of the Surgeon General, Department of the Army: *Textbook of Military Medicine Part 1: Warfare, Weaponry and the Casualty, Medical Aspects of Chemical and Biological Warfare*. United States of America, 1997.

Nerve Agents. Chemical substances that inhibit acety-cholinesterase (AChE) in the body, causing excess acety-choline (ACh) production, are known as nerve agents. The body responds to an exposure by increased secretions (saliva, tears, rhinorrhea, sweating), urination, miosis (pinpoint pupils), diarrhea and other gastrointestinal effects, fasciculation (uncontrolled twitching of the muscles), convulsions, and apnea. There is rapid onset of health effects with symptoms that mirror those of organophosphate exposures and poisonings.

Blister or Vesicant Agents. Chemical substances that cause burns and blistering of the skin, eyes, and tissues of the respiratory system are blister or vesicant agents. Systemic poisoning can occur if significant exposure occurs. You should anticipate a latent period between time of exposure to time of symptoms. Cellular damage will occur within 1 to 2 minutes of exposure but clinical effects of exposure will usually not be seen for 2 to 48 hours (generally within 2 to 8 hours). Symptoms can include, but are not limited to: irritation and blisters on the skin; conjunctivitis, corneal opacity, and damage in the eyes; and mild, upper respiratory signs or marked airway damage.

Blood Agents or Cyanides. These are highly toxic chemical substances with rapid onset of health effects (cyanides). At low doses, symptoms include anxiety, hyperventilation, vertigo, headache, and vomiting; at high-dose exposures, seizures begin within 30 seconds, respiratory arrest occurs within 3 to 5 minutes, and asystole occurs within 6 to 10 minutes.[11]

Choking or Pulmonary Agents. Chemical substances that cause severe irritation and damage to the tissue of the respiratory system comprise the subgroup of choking or pulmonary agents. The damage resulting from exposure can include pulmonary edema, congestive heart failure, and cardiac arrest. Prehospital care is usually limited to decontamination and supportive medical care such as checking ABCs, supplying oxygen, providing airway support, and limiting activity and movement of the patient. Because the clinical effects of phosgene may not present for hours after the exposure (other than the initial irritation that is sometimes experienced), monitoring patients for effects of exposure must be part of the emergency response system plan.

Irritants or Riot Control Agents. These are chemical substances that cause immediate onset of pain, burning, and irritation of the respiratory system, exposed mucous membranes, and skin. The effects are usually short-term and almost never fatal in healthy individuals.[9]

Biologic Weapons

Biologic terrorism is the use of bacteria, fungi, viruses, or toxins to induce disease or death upon humans, animals, or plant life. (Toxins may be considered more of a chemical weapon than a biologic weapon because of their chemical properties.) Use of biologic substances as weapons is not a new technique; history depicts several events where fighting groups attempted to poison each other or water and food supplies. The Mongols in the 1300s catapulted the corpses of plague victims into the city of Kaffa to infect the defenders.[2] The besieged town was rapidly devastated by disease. British and early American settlers gave Native Americans blankets that had been used by victims of smallpox. The resulting infections decimated the tribes, who had no defenses against the disease.[2]

In 1979 in Sverdlovsk, Russia, there was an accidental release of pulmonary anthrax that killed at least 66 humans living or working downwind of the biologic weapons facility.[12] In 1992, Russian President Boris Yeltsin finally confirmed that the epidemic originated from an accidental release and not from contaminated beef.[13] Now, with the current economic and political status of the countries that comprised the former Soviet Union, many intelligence analysts fear that bioweapons are being quietly sold to terrorist organizations via the black market.

In the United States, militia groups and individuals have attempted to acquire biologic agents, with some success. However, their use has been thwarted by the law enforcement community.

Biologic weapons have been described as the poor man's atomic bomb. It has also been said that if you can make beer, you can make biologic weapons. Although this is clearly an oversimplification, it is not entirely inaccurate. In fact, if you recall the outcome of the Aum Shinrikyos' story, you will remember that when Japanese authorities raided the cult's headquarters, they discovered approximately a liter of *botulinus* toxin that the cult had created. The real issue is not the creation or acquisition of the agents, which is relatively easy to do. Rather, it is the delivery system required to accurately aerosolize and disperse the substance in an effective manner that is the key to a successful attack by a rogue group.

Biologic terrorism is more difficult to identify than other forms of terrorism. Unlike chemical attacks, which are essentially in-your-face events, biologic attacks are slow-motion riots. If an attack is successful and effective, exposure occurs and affects multiple patients who are unaware of their condition. Over a period of 24 hours to 10 days, depending on the etiological agent, patients start to present with flu-like symptoms and get progressively sicker. The number of patients increases rapidly with the potential for a regional or international public health crisis. The 9-1-1 system will be overburdened and the healthcare system will be overwhelmed, potentially to the point of collapse. The demand for supplies such as ventilators and antibiotics will quickly outstrip the available resources. The widespread illness and death that this type event could generate will create significant and complex problems for the entire community.

It has been reported that if 110 lb of anthrax spores were sprayed in ideal conditions along a 1.5-mile track upwind from a city of 500,000, the result could be 24,000 deaths.[11] *Botulinus* toxin is 100,000 times more toxic than sarin, the nerve agent used by the Aum Shinrikyo.[9] Unfortunately, the emergency service community can do little to assist patients who have contracted anthrax. In most cases, EMS provides a supportive medical role, treating symptomatic patients with the ABCs, oxygen, and fluids.

Identifying such a biologic event may rest solely on early recognition by the medical community of patient trends (clinical presentation and complaints). With the lack of available monitoring equipment and an inability to rapidly recognize that a release has occurred, it is imperative that the health care community plan immediately how they intend to address the results of this type of terrorism.

The potency and widespread effect of a biologic weapon cannot be underestimated nor can the impact on the health care system be ignored. What follows is a brief review of the primary biologic substances used as weapons; signs and symptoms, diagnosis, treatment, prophylaxis, and decontamination procedures are summarized in **Table 21-2**.

Anthrax. Anthrax has become a recognizable term to the general public because of events that followed the September 11th attack on the World Trade Center. Anthrax is easily produced, occurs naturally in many parts of the world, and has spores that can remain viable for years. A single test tube of feed stock can produce a kilogram of anthrax in about 96 hours in a fermenter.[14] Anthrax has been called wool sorter's disease because of the high incidence of exposure in wool mills. Anthrax is a spore-forming organism that produces infection in patients via inhalation, ingestion, or absorption. Symptoms begin to develop within 1 to 6 days after exposure. Clinical presentation includes, but is not limited to, generalized body and muscle aches, cough, fever, and fatigue or lethargy. In a few days, symptoms appear to improve but the untreated patient will then rapidly develop severe dyspnea, shock, and death in 24 to 36 hours.[13] EMS providers should use universal precautions with patients who have been exposed to anthrax, as they should with any patient contact. There are no reported cases of person-to-person transmission, even among the most recent (October 2001) series of cases.[14]

Botulinus Toxin. The neurotoxin *botulinus* toxin is a product of the bacterium *Clostridium botulinum* that is also the disease source for botulism. *Botulinus* toxin is 15,000 times more toxic than the nerve agent VX.[11] Symptoms can begin as early as 24 to 36 hours after exposure but may take several days after inhalation. Botulinus toxin blocks both the conduction of nerve impulses at the neuromuscular junction and nerve receptors in the autonomic nervous system.[13] It prevents the release of the neurotransmitter Ach, creating muscle weakness and paralysis.[11] The patient can experience bulbar palsy (loss of function of nerves from the upper portion of the spinal cord) and descending paralysis (head-to-toe progression). Other signs and symptoms can include difficulty speaking and swallowing, blurred vision, dilated pupils, drooping eye lids, and diplopia. Advanced stages of exposure include continued descending paralysis, which will eventually affect the diaphragm and accessory muscle involvement followed by respiratory arrest. Patient care is mainly supportive and these patients most likely will require ventilator support.[11] An antitoxin exists but requires early recognition of the exposure to be effective.

Table 21-2 Biologic Threats

ANTHRAX

Signs and Symptoms: Incubation period is 1 to 6 days. Fever, malaise, fatigue, cough, and mild chest discomfort are followed by severe respiratory distress with dyspnea, diaphoresis, stridor, and cyanosis. Shock and death occur within 24 to 36 hours of severe symptoms.

Diagnosis: Physical findings are nonspecific. Possible widened mediastinum. Detectable by Gram stain of the blood and by blood culture in the course of illness.

Treatment: Although usually not effective after symptoms are present, high-dose antibiotic treatment with penicillin, ciprofloxacin, or doxycycline should be undertaken. Supportive therapy may be necessary.

Prophylaxis: A licensed vaccine is available for use by those considered at risk of exposure. Vaccine schedule is at 0, 2, and 4 weeks for initial series, followed by booster shots at 6, 12, and 18 months, and annually thereafter.

Decontamination: Secretion and lesion precautions should be practiced. After an invasive procedure or autopsy is performed, the instruments and area used should be thoroughly decontaminated with a sporicidal agent such as iodine or chlorine.

PLAGUE

Signs and Symptoms: *Pneumonic plague* has an incubation period of 2 to 3 days. High fever, chills, hemoptysis, toxemia, progressing rapidly to dyspnea, stridor and cyanosis. Death results from respiratory failure, circulatory collapse, and bleeding diathesis. *Bubonic plague* has an incubation period of 2 to 10 days. Malaise, high fever, and tender lymph nodes (buboes) may progress spontaneously to the septicemic form, and spread to the central nervous system, lungs, and elsewhere

Diagnosis: Clinical diagnosis. A presumptive diagnosis can be made by Gram or Wayson stain of lymph node aspirates, sputum, or cerebral spinal fluid. Plague can also be cultured.

CHOLERA

Signs and Symptoms: Incubation period is 1 to 5 days. Asymptomatic to severe with sudden onset. Vomiting, abdominal distention, and pain with little or no fever followed rapidly by diarrhea. Fluid losses may exceed 5 to 10 liters per day. Without treatment, death may result from severe dehydration, hypovolemia, and shock.

Diagnosis: Clinical diagnosis; watery diarrhea and dehydration. Microscopic examination of stool samples reveals few or no red or white cells. Cholera can be identified in stool by darkfield or phase contrast microscopy and can be grown on a variety of culture media.

Treatment: Fluid and electrolyte replacement. Antibiotics such as tetracycline, ampicillin, or trimethoprim-sulfamethoxazole will shorten the duration of diarrhea.

Prophylaxis: A licensed, killed vaccine is available but provides only about 50% protection and lasts no more than 6 months. Vaccination schedule is at 0 and 4 weeks, with booster doses every 6 months.

Decontamination: Personal contact rarely causes infection; however, enteric precautions and careful hand washing should be frequently employed. Bactericidal solutions such as hypochlorite would provide adequate decontamination.

TULAREMIA

Signs and Symptoms: *Ulceroglandular tularemia* presents with a local ulcer and regional lymphadenopathy, fever, chills, headache, and malaise. *Typhoidal* or *septicemic tularemia* presents with fever, headache, malaise, substernal discomfort, prostration, weight loss and a nonproductive cough.

Diagnosis: Clinical diagnosis; physical findings are usually nonspecific. Chest x-ray may reveal pneumonic process, mediastinal lymphadenopathy, or pleural effusion. Routine culture is possible but difficult. The diagnosis can be established by serology.

(Continued)

Table 21-2 Biologic Threats (Continued)

PLAGUE (Continued)

Treatment: Early administration of antibiotics is very effective. Supportive therapy is required for pneumonic and septicemic forms.

Prophylaxis: A licensed, killed vaccine is available. Initial dose is followed by a second, smaller dose 1 to 3 months later, and a third dose after another 3 to 6 months. A booster dose is given at 6, 12, and 18 months, and then every 1 to 2 years. This vaccine may not protect against aerosol exposure.

Decontamination: Secretion and lesion precautions with bubonic plague should be practiced. Strict isolation of patients with pneumonic plague. Heat, disinfectants, and exposure to sunlight render the bacteria harmless.

Q FEVER

Signs and Symptoms: Fever, cough, and pleuritic chest pain may occur as early as 10 days after exposure. Patients are not generally critically ill and the illness lasts from 2 days to 2 weeks.

Diagnosis: Q fever is not a clinically distinctive illness and may resemble a viral illness or other type of atypical pneumonia. The diagnosis is confirmed serologically.

Treatment: Q fever is generally a self-limiting illness even without treatment. Tetracycline or doxycycline are the treatments of choice and are orally administered for 5 to 7 days. Q fever endocarditis is rare and much more difficult to treat.

Prophylaxis: Treatment with tetracycline during the incubation period may delay but not prevent the onset of symptoms. An activated, whole-cell vaccine provides effective protection against exposure, but severe local reactions to this vaccine may be seen in those who already possess immunity.

Decontamination: Patients who are exposed to Q fever by aerosol do not present a risk for secondary contamination or re-aerosolization of the organism. Decontamination is accomplished with soap and water or a weak (0.5%) hypochlorite solutions.

TULAREMIA (Continued)

Treatment: Administration of antibiotics with early treatment is very effective.

Prophylaxis: A live, attenuated vaccine is available as an investigational new drug (IND). It is administered once by scarification. A 2-week course of tetracycline, administered after exposure, is effective as a prophylaxis.

Decontamination: Secretion and lesion precautions should be practiced. Strict isolation of patients is not required. Organisms are relatively easy to render harmless by heat and disinfectants.

SMALL POX

Signs and Symptoms: Clinical manifestation begins acutely with malaise, fever, rigors, vomiting, headache, and backache. Lesions appear 2 to 3 days later and quickly progress from macules to papules and eventually to pustular vesicles. They are more abundant on the extremities and face and develop synchronously.

Diagnosis: Tests of electron and light microscopy are not capable of discriminating *variola* from *vaccina*, monkeypox or cowpox. The new PCR diagnostic techniques may be more accurate in discriminating between *variola* and other orthopox viruses.

Treatment: At present there is no effective chemotherapy and treatment of a clinical case remains supportive.

Prophylaxis: Immediate vaccination or revaccination should be undertaken for all personnel exposed. Vaccinia-immune globulin (VIG) is of value in post-exposure prophylaxis of smallpox when given within the first week following exposure, and with vaccination.

Decontamination: Strict quarantine with respiratory isolation for a minimum of 16 to 17 days following exposure is required for all contacts. Patients should be considered infectious until all scabs separate.

(Continued)

Table 21-2 Biologic Threats (Continued)

VENEZUELAN EQUINE ENCEPHALITIS

Signs and Symptoms: Sudden onset of illness with general malaise, spiking fevers, rigors, severe headache, photophobia, and myalgias. Nausea, vomiting, cough, sore throat, and diarrhea may follow. Full recovery takes 1 to 2 weeks.

Diagnosis: Clinical diagnosis. Physical findings are usually non-specific. The white blood cell count often shows a striking leukopenia and lymphopenia. Virus isolation may be made from serum, and, in some cases, throat-swab specimens.

Treatment: Supportive therapy only.

Prophylaxis: A live, attenuated vaccine is available as an investigational new drug. A second, formalin-inactivated, killed vaccine is available for boosting antibody titers in those who initially received the live vaccine.

Decontamination: Blood and body fluid precautions, using body substance isolation (BSI) should be employed. Human cases are infectious for mosquitoes for at least 72 hours. The virus can be destroyed by heat (80°C/176°F for 30 minutes) and ordinary disinfectants.

VIRAL HEMORRHAGIC FEVERS

Signs and Symptoms: Viral hemorrhagic fevers (VHFs) are febrile illnesses which can be complicated by easy bleeding, petechiae, hypotension, shock, flushing of the face and chest, and edema. Constitutional symptoms such as malaise, myalgias, headache, vomiting, and diarrhea may occur in any hemorrhagic fevers.

Diagnosis: Clinical diagnosis; watery diarrhea and dehydration. Microscopic exam of stool samples reveals few or no red or white cells. Can be identified in stool by darkfield or phase contrast microscopy and can be grown on a variety of culture media.

Treatment: Intensive supportive care may be required. Antiviral therapy with ribavirin may be useful in several of these infections. Convalescent plasma may be effective in Argentine hemorrhagic fever.

Prophylaxis: The only licensed VHF vaccine is yellow fever vaccine. Prophylactic ribavirin may be effective for Lassa fever, Rift Valley fever, CCHF and possibly HFRS.

Decontamination: Decontaminate surfaces with hypochlorite or phenolic disinfectant. Isolation measures and barrier nursing procedures are indicated.

BOTULINUS TOXINS

Signs and Symptoms: Ptosis, generalized weakness, dizziness, dry mouth and throat, blurred vision and diplopia, dysarthia, dysphonia, and dysphagia, followed by symmetrical descending flaccid paralysis and development of respiratory failure. Symptoms can begin as early as 24 to 36 hours after inhalation of toxin, but may take several days.

Diagnosis: Clinical diagnosis. No routine laboratory findings. Bioterrorism or biowarfare should be suspected if numerous collocated casualties have progressive descending bulbar, muscular, and respiratory weakness.

Treatment: Intubation and ventilatory assistance for respiratory failure. Tracheostomy may be required. Administration of botulinus antitoxin (IND product) may prevent or decrease progression to respiratory failure and hasten recovery.

STAPHYLOCOCCAL ENTEROTOXIN B (SEB)

Signs and Symptoms: Sudden onset of fever, chills, headache, myalgia, and nonproductive cough from 3 to 12 hours after aerosol exposure. Some patients may develop shortness of breath and retrosternal chest pain. Fever may last 2 to 5 days, and cough may persist up to 4 weeks. Patients may also experience nausea, vomiting, and diarrhea if they swallow the toxin. Higher exposure levels can lead to septic shock and death.

Diagnosis: Clinical diagnosis; patient experiences a febrile respiratory syndrome without abnormalities appearing on chest x-rays. Large numbers of patients presenting with typical symptoms and signs of SEB pulmonary exposure would suggest an intentional attack.

Treatment: Treatment is limited to supportive care. Artificial ventilation might be needed for very severe cases, and attention to fluid management is essential.

(Continued)

Table 21-2 Biologic Threats (Continued)

BOTULINUS TOXINS (Continued)	STAPHYLOCOCCAL ENTEROTOXIN B (SEB) (Continued)
Prophylaxis: Pentavalent toxoid (types A, B, C, D, and E) is available as an IND product for those at high risk of exposure.	Prophylaxis: Use of protective mask. There is currently no vaccine available to prevent SEB infection.
Decontamination: Hypochlorite (0.5% solution for 10 to 15 minutes) and/or soap and water. Toxin is not dermally active and secondary aerosols are not a hazard from patients.	Decontamination: Hypochlorite (0.5% solution for 10 to 15 minutes) and/or soap and water. Destroy any food that may have been contaminated.
RICIN	**TRICHOTHECENE MYCOTOXINS (T2)**
Signs and Symptoms: Weakness, fever, cough, and hypothermia about 36 hours after aerosol exposure, followed in the next 12 hours by hypotension and cardiovascular collapse.	Signs and Symptoms: Exposure causes skin pain, pruritus, redness, vesicles, necrosis, and sloughing of epidermis. Effects on the airway include nose and throat pain, nasal discharge, itching and sneezing, cough, dyspnea, wheezing, chest pain, and hemoptysis. Toxin also produces effects after ingestion or eye contact. Severe poisoning results in prostration, weakness, ataxia, collapse, shock, and death.
Diagnosis: Signs and symptoms noted above in large numbers of geographically clustered patients could suggest an exposure to aerosolized ricin. The rapid time course to severe symptoms and death would be unusual for infectious agents. Laboratory findings are non-specific except for specific serum ELISA. Acute and convalescent sera should be collected.	Diagnosis: Should be suspected if an aerosol attack occurs in the form of "yellow rain" with droplets of yellow fluid contaminating clothes and the environment. Confirmation requires testing of blood, tissue, and environmental samples.
Treatment: Patient management is supportive. Presently there is no available antitoxin. Gastric decontamination measures should be employed if the toxin is ingested.	Treatment: There is no specific antidote. Superactivated charcoal should be given orally if the toxin was swallowed.
Prophylaxis: Presently there is no vaccine or prophylactic antitoxin available for human use. Use of a protective mask (respirator) is currently the best protection against inhalation if an attack/exposure is anticipated.	Prophylaxis: The only defense is to wear personal protective equipment during an attack. No specific immunotherapy or chemotherapy is available for use in the field.
Decontamination: Weak hypochlorite solutions and/or soap and water can decontaminate skin surfaces. Ricin is not volatile, so secondary aerosols are generally not a danger to health care providers.	Decontamination: Outer garments should be removed and exposed skin should be decontaminated with soap and water. Eye exposure should be treated by copious saline irrigation. Once decontamination is complete, isolation is not required.

Source: United States Army Medical Research Institute of Infectious Diseases: *Medical Management of Biological Casualties Handbook*, ed 2. Ft. Detrick, Fredrick, MD, 1996.

Cholera. The infectious disease cholera usually has a rapid onset in those who are exposed. Sudden nausea, vomiting, intestinal cramping, profuse watery diarrhea, and fatigue are characteristic of the disease. Patients with cholera can easily lose 5 to 10 liters of fluid a day, resulting in an electrolyte imbalance. Without treatment and stabilization, the patient may experience hypovolemia, shock, and death. Patient care generally consists of fluid and electrolyte replenishment.[2, 15]

Plague. An infectious disease usually found in the rodent population, plague is normally spread via the bites of infected fleas. It can also be spread through an intentional release and inhalation exposure. Plague normally appears in three forms: bubonic, primary septicemic, and pneumonic.[16]

Pneumonic plague has a reported mortality of 100%.[16] Pneumonic plague is the airborne form of the so-called black plague with accompanying symptoms that include fever, hemoptysis, and pathogenic lymph node destruction.[17] This form of plague is highly contagious, can be transmitted from person to person, and is rapidly fatal. Depending on the exposure dose, pneumonic plague will have a rapid onset after a 2- to 3-day incubation period. The pneumonia will progress rapidly, resulting in dyspnea, stridor, and cyanosis. As the disease process progresses, respiratory arrest, circulatory collapse, and an accompanying diathesis usually result.[13]

In bubonic plague, incubation periods can range from 2 to 10 days, followed by rapid onset of the disease. Clinical presentation includes fatigue or malaise, high-grade fever, and lymph node tenderness at one or more sites. The patient may also have purpuric and black necrotic lesions.[13]

Q Fever. First identified in Australia, Q fever gets its name from Query Fever because the causative agent was unknown. It would not be until 1937 that an organism, *Coxiella burnetii*, was identified as the responsible agent. *C burnetii* is highly contagious when spread by aerosolized inhalation and is resistant to heat and desiccation. A single inhaled organism may produce illness.[15]

After the usual incubation period Q fever manifests as a self-limiting febrile event that can last from 2 days to 2 weeks. General patient complaints includes fatigue, myalgias, headaches, and acute nondifferentiated febrile illness. In most instances, acute Q fever will resolve itself without antibiotic treatment.

Ricin. Ricin, a potent toxin, is a water-soluble derivative of the castor bean as well as a byproduct of the production of castor oil. The wash from preparing castor oil contains up to 5% ricin. As little as 1 mg can kill an exposed individual.[2,18] Castor beans are available globally and the derived toxin is relatively easy to produce.

When ricin is inhaled, patients can experience fatigue, weakness, cough, and chest tightness within 4 to 8 hours after the exposure. Severe respiratory distress, pulmonary edema, and cardiac arrest from hypoxemia will occur within 36 to 72 hours. Patient care is supportive, with a special focus on managing the pulmonary edema. Patients suspected of ingesting the substance would experience nausea, vomiting, severe diarrhea, gastrointestinal hemorrhage, and necrosis of the liver, spleen, and kidneys. Shock and death would occur within 3 days. Patient treatment includes providing airway support and oxygen; gastric lavage, superactivated charcoal, and additional pharmacological intervention may also be required.[11,13,15]

Smallpox. The last natural case of smallpox was seen in 1977, and the World Health Organization (WHO) declared the disease eradicated in 1980, primarily because of vaccinations. Two WHO-sanctioned repositories of the smallpox virus (*variola* virus) remain: one at the Centers for

Disease Control and Prevention (CDC) in Atlanta, Georgia, and the other at a similar facility called Vector in Novizbersk, Russia. However, the number of clandestine stockpiles that exist continues to be speculative and unverified.[11,15] As events in the Middle East, and specifically in Iraq, have shown, it is difficult to project whether rogue nations, organizations, and individuals possess this virus. Possession and continued production of the smallpox virus directly violates the January 1996 recommendation by the WHO that all smallpox inventories be destroyed by 1999.

Smallpox is infectious as an aerosol, is highly contagious, and has a high mortality rate. Smallpox symptoms will generally present within 7 to 17 days of exposure. Symptoms include fatigue, general muscle and back pain, fever, headache, and vomiting. Within 48 to 72 hours, the patient may develop a pox-like rash on the face, upper arms, and lower extremities, which progresses to the body trunk over subsequent days. Approximately 30% of exposed individuals become ill, making smallpox less contagious than influenza, measles, and tuberculosis. Treatment of the smallpox patient is supportive and the patient must be quarantined for at least 17 days, until scab healing is complete.[11]

Staphylococcal Enterotoxin B (SEB). *Staphylococcal enterotoxin B* (SEB) results from improperly stored or handled food. SEB characteristics vary, depending on whether the virus was ingested or inhaled. A patient who ingested SEB can experience nausea, vomiting, and diarrhea with substantial fluid loss. Inhalation patients can experience an acute onset of high-grade fever, chills, headaches, myalgias, and nonproductive coughing within 3 to 12 hours of exposure.[13] In severe cases, dyspnea and retrosternal chest pain can develop. Prolonged fevers of 103° to 106°F, with varying chills and exhaustion, may continue for up to 5 days. A physical examination of this patient will probably be unremarkable, but extreme or advanced cases may develop severe pulmonary problems such as atelectasis, pulmonary edema, or Adult Respiratory Distress Syndrome (ARDS).

Treatment of SEB-poisoned patients is limited to supportive care, including airway support, oxygen, and fluid replenishment.

Trichothecene Mycotoxins (T2). Trichothecene mycotoxins (T2) are more than 40 toxins produced by a variety of fungi. T2 ingestion results in vomiting, skin lesions, hemorrhage, skin pain, pruritus, redness, vesicles, and eventual sloughing of the epidermis. Respiratory effects include nasal and throat pain, nasal itching, sneezing and discharge, dyspnea, hemoptysis, and chest pain. High-dose exposure can result in the development of rapid-onset circulatory shock, lactic acidosis, and death within 12 to 24 hours. Symptoms can be confused with sepsis or radiation sickness, so an accurate and thorough history is needed for proper diagnosis. T2 is the only dermally active toxin that presents a secondary exposure threat to unprotected responders; use universal precautions. Contact with the substance can cause blistering and, at times, has been confused with exposure to mustard gas.

Tularemia. Tularemia (also known as rabbit fever and deer fly fever) is a zoonotic disease. It is a hardy bacterium that can survive for weeks in carcasses, hides, soil, or water. Cases have been reported where the bacterium has survived for years in frozen rabbit meat.[15] Application of disinfectants or heat can kill tularemia.

Humans acquire the disease usually as a result of inoculation with blood or tissue fluids from an infected source (infected animals, deerflies, mosquitoes, or ticks).[15] An infrequent exposure is by inhaling or ingesting contaminated dust, food, or water. Inhalation of only 10 to 50 organisms can cause disease in humans.[11,15]

After an incubation period that ranges from 2 to 10 days, patients experience an acute onset of fever, chills, headaches, myalgias, and nonproductive coughing. The inhaled tularemia causes typhoidal tularemia that often has a pneumonic component.[15] Tularemia has a 100% infection rate for those who are exposed but less than a 4% mortality.[11] Treatment consists of supportive care and antibiotic intervention.

Venezuelan Equine Encephalitis (VEE). Venezuelan equine encephalitis (VEE) is a highly infectious virus with an almost 100% infection rate of exposed individuals, but only a 1% mortality rate. VEE is characterized by inflammation of the meninges and the brain itself, which accounts for the prevalence of central nervous system (CNS) symptoms in those who are exposed. VEE is acute in onset, exhausting, and short in duration.[15]

Symptoms of VEE exposure develop within 1 to 5 days and include photophobia, severe headaches, spiking fevers up to 104°F, generalized muscle and body aches, nausea, vomiting, diarrhea, and vigorous chills.[11] Increased CNS disease manifestations will be brought on by an aerosolized exposure. Patient care is supportive, consisting of ABCs, airway maintenance, and fluid replenishment where required.

Viral Hemorrhagic Fever (VHF). Viral Hemorrhagic Fevers (VHF) are caused by RNA viruses from several viral families. VHFs include Crimean-Congo hemorrhagic fever, Dengue fever, Ebola, Hantaviruses, and yellow fever, to name but just a few.

VHFs are febrile illnesses that are often complicated by ease of bleeding, edema, and postural hypotension. Other signs and symptoms include headache, photophobia, exhaustion, nausea, vomiting, diarrhea, altered mental state, capillary leaks, abdominal pain, vertigo, prominent fever, renal failure, and shock.[11,13] VHFs are moderately contagious and very often fatal.[19] Patient care is supportive with a focus on maintaining respiratory and hemodynamic status.

Summary

As the frequency of terrorist events in the United States increases, the past levels of security and safety we enjoyed are most likely gone. The complexities of responding to an act of terrorism are many; the need to be prepared is great. This chapter is not a solution to your organization's response to terrorism problems, but rather a prompt for

Remember:

In all patient contacts, especially with those suspected of contagious diseases, use of universal precautions is imperative for the safety of the responder!

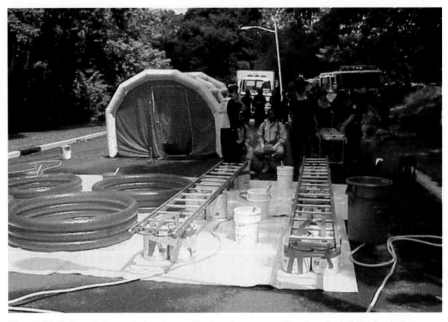

Figure 21-6 Preparation and planning are the keys to success. *(Courtesy Paul M. Maniscalco)*

serious discussions about the issues you and your organization will confront. Heightening the awareness levels within your emergency response organization, participating in the available training, executing internal policy, conducting exercises, and procuring the required personal protective equipment and response assets are just the start (**Figure 21-6**).

Contemporary terrorism is bringing continual changes in technique and execution. Clearly, the need for individuals and organizations to stay current is a must. There are numerous training programs and reference resources that are available to assist you with this endeavor. Stay current—stay safe!

Appendix A

Incidents

On January 30, 2002, two San Diego, California medics were injured when a patient became combative while being transported to the hospital. The patient broke loose from the stretcher kicking a paramedic in the face. The male patient then entered the cab where he placed the driver in a choke hold. The ambulance veered off of the highway striking some shrubs.

Two Pike County, Indiana, medics were found dead in their station on April 19, 2001, by coworkers. A third Pike County EMT was arrested for the shooting.[1]

On December 2, 2001, a Detroit firefighter was on night watch and went outside to check on a noise in the station's parking lot where he was shot twice by an unknown assailant. He survived thanks to his fellow firefighters' fast actions.

On October 29, 2001, Security Village Fire Department, Colorado firefighter went to investigate a strange noise outside of Station 2. Someone approached the firefighter from behind and stabbed him in the abdomen. The firefighter was released from the hospital the following day with only minor injuries.

A Philadelphia paramedic was pistol whipped by his own partner on May 27, 2001, while enroute to a call.

A 35-year-old woman was shot and killed in the Campbellsport Fire Department, Wisconsin, station on January 6, 2001. The woman, a member of the Department, was shot five times by her ex-boyfriend, also a firefighter in the station.[2]

Memphis, Tennessee, firefighters who responded to a house fire on March 8, 2000, were ambushed by one of their own. The suspect, also a Memphis firefighter, had just returned to work "after an extended leave on disability."[3] A responding Shelby County Sheriff's Deputy was shot and killed as he drove into the scene. His car crashed through a fence. The suspect was shot when he refused to put down the weapon.

Two Memphis paramedics were assaulted on February 14, 2000. The medics were in their unit treating the victim of a beating when the rear window was shattered and a gunman broke into the patient compartment. The gunman began beating the victim as he lay on the stretcher. The medics and the patient were able to escape.[4]

An Oakland, California, police sergeant and paramedics were fired upon by an unknown assailant as they attempted to treat the victim of a shooting. The incident occurred on December 26, 1999. Neither the sergeant nor the medics were injured.[5]

A pipe bomb was found beneath a Parkwood Volunteer Fire Department ambulance on December 11, 1999. The ambulance was dispatched with fire units to a kitchen fire in Durham County, North Carolina. The device was found by a crew member who was returning to the unit. It consisted of a battery, shotgun shell, nails, gunpowder, and firecrackers. A teenage boy was questioned about the device.[6]

While attempting to enter an apartment to assist an elderly woman back into bed, a five-year veteran of Ocala Fire Rescue (Florida) was shot in the chest. The October 21, 1999, incident occurred when the EMT attempted to enter the apartment through a rear window. He was actually entering an adjoining apartment where the 69-year-old occupant thought he was being burglarized. The shooting occurred while the elderly man was on the phone with 911 reporting the burglary.[7]

A Spartanburg County (South Carolina) EMS paramedic was shot once in the face by a woman in May 1999. The woman reportedly became upset that she could not be transported to a hospital in Atlanta, Georgia. She walked away, returned with a .38-caliber handgun, and shot the medic between the upper lip and the nose. The bullet lodged a short distance from the spine (Maniscalco P, personal communication with Don Lundy, 1999).

In Montgomery County, Maryland, a paramedic was stabbed in the throat and under the arm. The unit had responded to a sick person on August 8, 1998. They arrived to find a man on the porch of a house. As the patient became violent, the medics attempted to retreat and the stabbing occurred.[8]

Two firefighters in Conneaut, Ohio, stopped traffic to allow an ambulance to back out of a driveway. A motorist sped through, shooting the firefighters; one was struck in the head.[9]

Two Toledo, Ohio, firefighters were injured on February 13, 1998, when a gunman went on a rampage that left three people dead and four injured. As one ambulance transported a wounded 10-year-old child, the suspect stepped in front of the unit and fired one shotgun blast into its windshield. The unit's driver was injured by the flying glass that struck his head and eyes. A lieutenant driving a second unit ran to aid the firefighter. A second blast struck the lieutenant's arm, chest, and abdomen.[11]

During a fire in a Taylor County, Florida, greenhouse, a .22-caliber rifle overheated and discharged. A firefighter was struck in the chest and died on October 22, 1997.[11]

A Moapa Valley, Nevada, volunteer fire chief responding to a medical emergency on October 21, 1997, was injured when the patient became extremely combative. The chief, who was pushed and fell during the scuffle, was treated for a broken ankle and released.[12]

Five shots were fired at a New York City ambulance transporting a patient in cardiac arrest to Kings County Hospital in Brooklyn. No one was injured in the February 22, 1997, incident. The ambulance was struck only once.[13]

A Washington, D.C., firefighter was shot on December 9, 1996, while transporting a shooting victim to the hospital. The unit had stopped so that medics could insert an IV line. Two men began shooting at the ambulance, striking it at least eight times. The firefighter was struck in the leg. The original patient was struck in the ambush and later died.[14]

Four fire officers were shot to death on April 24, 1996, by a disgruntled Jackson, Mississippi, firefighter in their headquarters building.[15]

On Christmas Day in 1994, two Philadelphia paramedics were attacked by a knife-wielding assailant. The medics had been stopped by two men on the street while the unit was responding to another call. One man lying on the ground, thought to be injured, jumped up and began swinging a knife at the medics and screaming that he wanted their drug bag. Both were treated at a local hospital for their wounds.[16]

Responding to a false report of a gas leak, three firefighters were injured when a Molotov cocktail was thrown into the cab of FDNY Engine 93. They were burned over 50% of their bodies. This incident on July 9, 1993, followed a police incident the previous night in a Washington Heights neighborhood.[17]

Denver firefighters responded to assist police with a possible suicide on January 31, 1993. Attempting to check on the victim, they put a ladder up to the second floor. As one firefighter ascended the ladder he was shot in the neck by the suicidal man. He died later at a local hospital. The gunman eventually did commit suicide.[18]

The Los Angeles riots were tragic for one Los Angeles City firefighter. On April 29, 1992, an LA city ladder truck was responding to a fire when a car pulled beside the unit. One occupant of the vehicle shot into the cab and struck the driver of the ladder truck in the face. He was transported to a local hospital on the truck. The bullet severed his carotid artery and lodged in his neck partially paralyzing the firefighter.[19]

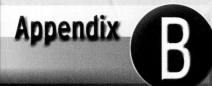

Soft Body Armor

Concern for the safety of emergency service personnel in the United States is increasing. The weapons used on the street today have changed drastically from those used several years ago. In the past, street people used Saturday-night specials, little, small-caliber handguns, often held together by bailing wire or tape. Today, these people are armed with sophisticated weapons that range from small, 9-mm pistols to compact, automatic-assault weapons. Because of the growing use of these deadly weapons, fire protection agencies, individual firefighters, and EMS personnel are realizing the importance of using soft body armor.

In Houston, Texas, ambulances are equipped with soft body armor for firefighter paramedics.[1] The Los Angeles City Fire Department has equipped each piece of apparatus, including Battalion Chief vehicles, with soft body armor.

Catalogs advertising collectibles, uniforms, books, and training materials mailed to fire service personnel now include advertisements for soft body armor.[2] Publishers of law enforcement periodicals, which have featured soft body armor ads for years, are now including fire and EMS professionals on their unsolicited mailing lists.[3]

Violence toward fire, rescue, and EMS personnel continues to escalate. Individuals, as well as entire departments, will probably purchase soft body armor in the future. Knowing its construction and protection qualities will help you to decide what type of equipment to purchase.

Contrary to popular belief, Kevlar is not bulletproof, but it is recognized as the preferred material for bullet- and fragment-resistant protective apparel (Miner LH: Ballistic Testing of Used Soft Body Armor of Kevlar Aramid, Wilmington, Del, 1987, EI Du Pont De Nemours & Co, Industrial Fibers Division, photocopy). It was introduced in 1972 by E.I. Du Pont De Nemours and Company. Since that time, it has been blended with natural cloth and synthetic material to produce work uniforms and protective clothing for emergency service workers. An ounce of Kevlar is 5 times stronger than an ounce of steel, extremely stretch-resistant, inherently flame-resistant, and will not melt.[4]

A bullet striking any object produces energy. When a bullet strikes a Kevlar vest, the fibers surrounding the point of impact absorb and dissipate the initial shock of the bullet over a large area, thus preventing the projectile from penetrating the material and reducing the possibility of blunt trauma (**Figure B-1**). Bruises, lacerations, and some internal injuries may occur if you are struck by a bullet or fragments while wearing soft body armor. If you are shot while wearing soft body armor, you must be examined at a medical facility.

Not all body armor is equally strong. It is classified into six levels of protection. The threat level chart shown is offered only as a guideline.

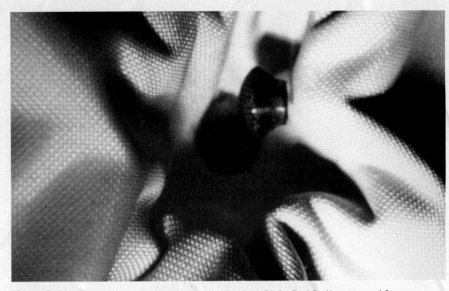

Figure B-1 Bullet bouncing off soft body armor. *(Courtesy E.I. Du Pont De Nemours and Company, Wilmington, DE)*

Before you purchase any soft body armor, you must know the type of weapons being used on the street.[5] Keep abreast of this changing information and adjust your level of protection accordingly. In all instances, make sure the body armor you purchase meets or exceeds the specifications required by the current National Institute of Justice Standard No. 0101.03.

Adjusting to the feel of wearing body armor takes time. New vests may feel bulky at first. During summer months, expect to feel hot and somewhat uncomfortable. Remember that the vest is giving you added protection, and any discomfort you may experience is a small price to pay for this protection.

Specific instructions for the care of your body armor are provided by the manufacturer. However, the following guidelines apply to all brands:

- Hand wash the body armor in cold water with a mild detergent.
- Thoroughly rinse and remove all detergent. (An improperly rinsed vest can develop reduced stopping power.)
- Never use bleach or any product containing bleach.
- Never dry clean. (Check manufacturer's specifications.)
- Never machine wash or machine dry.
- Always drip-dry indoors.
- Return the vest to the manufacturer for repairs.[6]

Inspect your body armor regularly. Look for signs of abrasion, fabric fraying, or unraveling. A washed-out appearance or permanent wrinkles indicate unusual wear. Ensure that the vest fits properly and is relatively comfortable. Armor should be replaced after it has stopped a bullet or after 5 years of normal use. Do not abuse the vest; treat it as if your life depends on it, because it does.

Table B-1 Threat Level Chart

Threat Level	Ballistic Protection
I	.22-caliber long rifle handgun rounds .38-caliber special projectiles
IIA	.22-caliber long rifle handgun rounds .38-caliber special projectiles .357 Magnum 158 grain striking at 1250 ft/sec 9 mm 124 grain striking at 1090 ft/sec
II	.22-caliber long rifle handgun rounds .38-caliber special projectiles .357 Magnum 158 grain striking at 1250 ft/sec .357 Magnum 158 grain striking at 1395 ft/sec 9 mm 124 grain striking at 1090 ft/sec 9 mm 124 grain striking at 1175 ft/sec
IIIA	.22-caliber long rifle handgun rounds .38-caliber special projectiles .357 Magnum 158 grain striking at 1250 ft/sec .357 Magnum 158 grain striking at 1395 ft/sec 9 mm 124 grain striking at 1090 ft/sec 9 mm 124 grain striking at 1175 ft/sec .977 124 grain striking at 1400 ft/sec .44 Magnum semi wad cutter striking at 1400 ft/sec
III	.22-caliber long rifle handgun rounds .38-caliber special projectiles .357 Magnum 158 grain striking at 1250 ft/sec .357 Magnum 158 grain striking at 1395 ft/sec 9 mm 124 grain striking at 1090 ft/sec 9 mm 124 grain striking at 1175 ft/sec .977 124 grain striking at 1400 ft/sec .44 Magnum semi wad cutter striking at 1400 ft/sec 7.62 mm (308 Winchester)
IV	.22-caliber long rifle handgun rounds .38-caliber special projectiles .357 Magnum 158 grain striking at 1250 ft/sec .357 Magnum 158 grain striking at 1395 ft/sec 9 mm 124 grain striking at 1090 ft/sec 9 mm 124 grain striking at 1175 ft/sec .977 124 grain striking at 1400 ft/sec .44 Magnum semi wad cutter striking at 1400 ft/sec 7.62 mm (308 Winchester) 30.06 projectiles

Notes

Preface

[1]Scott F: Caught in the Crossfire, Advance for Respiratory Therapists. Jan. *Advance for Respiratory Therapists* January 1989.

[2]Gaston B: Caught in the Crossfire, *Jems* 1993;18:75.

Chapter 1

[1]News and Trends, *Fire Chief* 1989;33(3):12.

[2]American Body Armor & Equipment, Inc: Advertisement for second-generation, light-weight body armor. *Emergency Medical Services* 1987;16(3):61.

[3]Protection Development International Corp: Antiterrorist cab (advertisement). *Fire Chief* 1988;32(8):66.

Chapter 2

[1]Cab forward apparatus does not protect personnel in the front seat with the engine block, but no matter what type of cab you are using, follow the same positioning procedures.

Chapter 3

[1]Description of a vehicle with steel-plating, gun ports, bullet-proof glass and tires, tear-gas launchers, and an oil tank that dumps oil on the roadway when activated. Arizona Department of Public Safety: *Criminal Intelligence Information Bulletin* 1988;88–07.

Chapter 4

[1]US Department of Justice, Federal Bureau of Investigation: Uniform crime reports, 1986 in *Federal Bureau of Investigation Pub No 181-487:60532*. Washington, DC, US Government Printing Office, 1987.

[2]Adams RJ, McTernan TM, Remsberg C: *Street Survival*, Northbrook, IL, Calibre Press, 1987.

[3]Detecting Concealed Firearms, Part 1. *Calibre Press Street Survival Newsline* [online news service]. 1998;304.

[4]Maryland State Police troopers wear Stetson uniform hats that are similar to those worn by military drill instructors.

Chapter 5

[1]Fire Specialist Bruce A. Snyder, Baltimore County Fire Department, is a former member of the Baltimore City Fire Department where he was assigned to Truck 12. On the night of 8 September 1982, he was detailed to Engine 46. He was one of the firefighters on the scene of this incident. (Krebs DR, personal communication with Snyder BA, 1988)

Chapter 6

[1]Incledon PJ: Know the risk: window entry *With New York Firefighters* 1988;49(2):22.

Chapter 7

[1]Fite R, Sauer E: "1 Dead, 2 Injured." *The Sentinel* May 30, 1987.

[2]Fite R, Strong K: "Second Victim of Shooting Dies." *The Sentinel* June 3, 1987.

[3]Thompson GJ, Jenkins JB: *Verbal Judo, The Gentle Art of Persuasion.* New York, William Morrow and Co, Inc, 1993, pp 47–54.

[4]Ibid, p 130.

Chapter 8

[1]Adams RJ, McTernan TM, Remsberg C: *Street Survival.* Northbrook, IL, Calibre Press, 1987.

Chapter 9

[1]San Diego Fire Department: *McDonald's Restaurant Critique.* San Diego, CA, San Diego Fire Department, 1984.

Chapter 10

[1]Remsberg C: *The Tactical Edge.* Northbrook, Ill, Calibre Press, 1987.

[2]Fuselier GW: A practical overview of hostage negotiations, *FBI Law Enforcement Bulletin* 1981;50:2.

[3]Fuselier, p 2.

[4]Strentz T: A hostage psychological survival guide. *FBI Law Enforcement Bulletin* 1978; 47(11):1.

[5]Kobetz, p 80.

[6]Strentz, p 3.

[7]Bolz Jr FA: *How to be a Hostage and Live.* Secaucus, NJ, Lyle Stuart, Inc, 1987.

[8]Bolz, p 13.

[9]Strentz T: Law enforcement policy and ego defense of the hostage. *FBI Law Enforcement Bulletin* 1979;48(4):7.

[10]Fuselier, p 6.

Chapter 11

[1]US Department of Justice, Office of Justice Programs: *A Guide for Explosion and Bombing Scene Investigation.* Washington, DC, US Government Printing Office, 2000, p 3.

[2]Bombing Incidents, p 7.

[3]Stoffel J: *Explosives and Homemade Bombs.* ed 2. Illinois, Charles C. Thomas, 1972, p 36.

[4]Lenz RR: *Explosives and Bomb Disposal Guide.* Illinois, Charles C. Thomas, 1971, p 16.

[5]Stoffel, p 36.

[6]Morris C: Explosive Situation. *Police Magazine* 1996;9:48.

[7]US Department of Transportation: *Emergency Response Guidebook.* Available at *http://hazmat.dot.gov.*

[8]Morris, p 70.

[9]Smith A: Firefighting Today. *Firehouse Magazine* 1991;16(7):48.

[10]Bombing Incidents, p 23.

Chapter 12

[1]Beaty J: Tales of the Crank Trade. *Time* April 24, 1989.

[2]US Department of Justice: *DEA Meth Lab Seizures National Totals.* Available at: *http://www.usdoj.gov/dea/stats/drugstats.htm#meth.*

[3]US Department of Justice: *DEA Briefing Book.* Available at: *http://www.usdoj.gov/dea/briefingbook/page16-31.htm.*

[4]Koch Crime Institute: *Fast Facts About Meth.* Available at: *http://www.kci.org/meth_info/meth_facts.htm.*

[5]*DEA Briefing Book.*

[6]Molino LN: Clandestine drug labs part 1: what's brewing. *The Pennsylvania Fireman* 1989;52(5):60.

[7]Frye M: Clandestine Drug Labs and the First Responder. *Speaking of Fire* 1988;Winter:2.

[8]Firehouse.com. Hazardous Materials—Clandestine Drug Labs page. Available at: *http://www.firehouse.com/training/hazmat/2001/08_drug.html.*

[9]Lerario R, Methamphetamine Activity in the MAGLOCLEN Region. *Middle Atlantic-Great Lakes Organized Crime Law Enforcement Network:* 2000;April:4.

[10]Drug Enforcement Administration: MDMA—Ecstasy. *Drug Intelligence Brief* 1999;DEA-99019:4.

[11]Drug Enforcement Administration: Overview of Club Drugs. *Drug Intelligence Brief* 2000;DEA-20005:2.

[12]Perkins S: *Drug Identification Designer and Club Drugs.* Carrollton, TX, Alliance Press, 1999, p 5.

[13]Ibid, p 6.

[14]Ibid, p 3.

[15]Ibid, p 3.

[16]Maryland State Police: GHB and GBL, date rape drugs. *Maryland Intelligence Alert* 4(7):1.

Chapter 15

[1]US Fire Administration, Federal Emergency Management Agency: Wanton violence at Columbine High School. *USFA-TR-128* 1999;April:1.

[2]Ibid, p 10.

[3]ABCnews.com. Arsenal Found, Columbine-Style Threat Shuts Down California Campus page. Available at: *http://ABCnews.com.* Accessed January 30, 2001.

Chapter 16

[1]Osterburg JW: *Criminal Investigation, A Method for Reconstructing the Past*. Cincinnati, OH, Anderson Publishing Co, 1992, p 490.

[2]Fisher B: *Techniques of Crime Scene Investigation*, ed 4. New York, NY, Elsevier Science Publishing Co, Inc, 1987, p 6.

[3]Geberth VJ: *Practical Homicide Investigation*, ed 3. Florida, CRC Press, Inc, 1996, p 5.

[4]Ibid, p 536.

[5]Ibid, p 511.

[6]DiMaio V: *Gunshot Wounds, Practical Aspects of Firearms Ballistics, and Forensic Techniques*. Florida, CRC Press, Inc, 1993, p 36.

[7]Geberth, p 284.

[8]DiMaio, p 67.

[9]Geberth, p 287.

[10]Ibid, p 293.

[11]DiMaio, p 53.

[12]Ibid, p 57.

[13]Fisher, p 460.

[14]DiMaio, p 70.

[15]Fisher, p 342.

[16]Schiro G: *Collection and Preservation of Evidence*. Available at: *http://www.crime-scene-investigator.net/evidenc3.html*.

[17]Frickle LB: *Traffic Accident Reconstruction*. Chicago, IL, Northwestern University Traffic Institute, 1990.

Chapter 17

[1]Bureau of Justice Assistance: *Addressing Community Gang Problems: A Practical Guide*. Washington, DC, Bureau of Justice Assistance, 1998, p 19.

[2]Howell J: *Youth Gangs: An Overview. Juvenile Justice Bulletin*. Washington, DC, Office of Juvenile Justice and Delinquency Prevention, 1998, p 8.

[3]Ibid, p 1.

[4]Office of Juvenile Justice and Delinquency Prevention, US Department of Justice: *1998 National Youth Gang Survey*. Washington, DC, US Government Printing Office, 2000, p 12.

[5]*Calibre Press Street Survival Newsline* [online news service] 1997;288.

[6]Bureau of Justice Assistance, p 9.

[7]*1998 National Youth Gang Survey*, p 10.

[8]Landre R, Miller M, Porter D: *Gangs: A Handbook for Community Awareness*. New York, Facts on File, Inc, 1977, p 30.

[9]*Calibre Press Street Survival Newsline* [online news service] 1997;173.

[10]Landre, p 71.

[11]Office of Juvenile Justice and Delinquency Prevention, United States Department of Justice: *Gang Members on the Move*. Washington, DC, US Government Printing Office, 1998, p 2.

[12]Brantley A, DiRosa A: Gangs A National Perspective. *FBI Law Enforcement Bulletin* 1994;May:2.

[13]Landre, p. 78.

[14]*Calibre Press Street Survival Newsline* [online news service] 1996;6.

[15]Landre, p 77.

[16]The Mexican Mafia is a prison gang that originated in the California Division of Corrections.

[17]Macko S: ERRI Special Report: How Street Gangs Control Prisons. *ERRI Emergency Services Report* May 12, 1997.

[18]Denney J: Insider Threat: Political Threat to Local and National U.S. Interest, The Evolution and Emergency of "The Gang State." *ERRI Emergency Services Report* September 6, 1997.

[19]*Calibre Press Street Survival Newsline* [online news service] 1997;171:3.

[20]Landre, p 70.

[21]Street Gang Dynamics. The Coroner's Report, Information and Resources on Gang Intervention and Prevention page. Available at: *http://www.gangwar.com/dynamics.htm*. Accessed in 1997.

[22]Landre, p 76.

[23]Landre, p 77.

[24]*Calibre Press Street Survival Newsline* [online news service] 1997; 170:1.

[25]Landre p 84.

[26]Landre p 86.

[27]National Alliance of Gang Investigators Associations. The Motorcycle Gangs or Motorcycle Mafia? page. Available at: *http://www.nagia.org/Motorcycle_Gangs.htm*.

[28]Valdez A: Decoding the Secret Messages on the Wall. *Police* 1996; 20(4):31.

Chapter 18

[1]The phrase *less lethal* does not imply that the device is non-lethal.

[2]James S: Testing and Evaluating Less-Lethal Projectiles. *The Tactical Edge*. 1997;Spring:12.

[3]Edwards SM, Granfield J, Onnen J: Evaluation of Pepper Spray. National Institute of Justice, 1997, p 1.

[4]Epstein P, Fine J, Hu H: Tear Gas-Harassing Agent or Toxic Chemical Weapon? *JAMA* 1989;262(5):661.

[5]James S: Chemical Agents: Barricade Resolution Through Space Deprivation. *The Tactical Edge* 1998;Fall:30.

[6]James, p 37.

[7]Edwards, p 2–3.

[8]Science and Technology. *International Chiefs of Police* 1994;March:2.

[9]Counter Narcotics & Terrorism Operational Medical Support. The CONTOMS Dispatch page. Available at: *http://www.usuhs.mil/ccr/ccr.html*. Accessed July 1995.

[10]Hubbs K: Less Lethal Munitions, Are They Really Safe and Effective? *The Law Enforcement Trainer* 1998; July/August:14.

[11]Steele D: Less Than Lethal. *Law and Order* 1995:3.

[12]Campbell JE: *Basic Trauma Life Support, Advanced.* New Jersey, Prentice Hall, Inc, 1998, p 17.

[13]Hubbs, p 12.

[14]James, p 12..

Chapter 19

[1]Federal Emergency Management Agency, United States Fire Administration: *Civil Unrest, Recommendations for Organization and Operations During Civil Disturbances, Report of the Joint Fire/Police Task Force on Civil Unrest, FA-142.* Washington, DC, US Government Printing Office, 1994, p 9.

[2]Ibid.

Chapter 20

[1]McCauley D: Gasping for Breath. *Police* 1996;July:59.

[2]Cowen A: In a Bind. *Emergency Medical Services* 1995;June:54–58.

[3]Stratton S, Rogers C, Green K: Sudden Death in Individuals in Hobble Restraints During Paramedic Transport. *Annals of Emergency Medicine* 1995;May:7–11.

[4]United States Court of Appeals for the Fourth Circuit. *Melendez v. Howard County Government.* August 1997, p 1–8.

[5]United States District Court. *Price v. County of San Diego.* 990 Federal Supplement, January 1998, p 1236.

[6]Ibid, p 1238.

[7]Ibid, p 1238.

Chapter 21

[1]King K: "Alleged plot involved Anthrax, HIV and Rabies." *The Brownsville Herald* July 14, 1998.

[2]Christen HT, Maniscalco PM: *Understanding Terrorism and Managing Its Consequence,* ed 2. Upper Saddle River, NJ, Prentice Hall/Brady Publishing, 2001.

[3]FBI. Available at: *http://www.fbi.gov/lab/bomsum/eubdc.htm.*

[4]The Congressional Record. The US Senate Judiciary Hearings on Terrorism, September 3, 1998 page. Available at: *http://www.access.gpo.gov/su_docs/aces/aces150.html.*

[5]The Congressional Record. The Global Proliferation of Weapons of Mass Destruction, Hearings before the Permanent Subcommittee on Investigations, US Senate, March 13, 20 and 22, 1996 page. Available at *http://www.access.gpo.gov/su_docs/aces/aces150.html.*

[6]Maniscalco PM: Domestic Preparedness: The Grand Illusion Emergency Medical Services. *The Journal of Emergency Medical Care, Rescue and Transportation* 2001; 30 (4).

[7]US Army Medical Research Institute of Chemical Defense: *Medical Management of Chemical Casualties Handbook,* ed 2. Aberdeen MD, Chemical Casualty Care Office, 1995.

[8]Staten C: Houston chemical incidents today; similar to those in New Orleans, Florida. Emergencynet News page. Available at: *http://www.emergencynet.com/main.htm.* Accessed July 8, 1998.

[9]FEMA: *HMEP Guidelines for Public Sector Hazardous Materials Training (1998).* Document available at *http://www.usfa.fema.gov/hazmat/hmep/HMEPIntro.pdf.*

[10]US Department of Transportation, Research and Special Programs Administration: Transport Canada, Safety and Security, Dangerous Goods; Mexico Secretariat of Transportation and Communications, *1996 North American Emergency Response Guidebook.* Washington, DC, 1996.

[11]US Army: CBDCOM Domestic Preparedness Program. Washington DC, 1997.

[12]Meselson M, Guillemin J, Hugh-Jones M, et al: The Sverdlovsk Anthrax Outbreak of 1979. *Science* 1994;266:1202–1208.

[13]Office of the Surgeon General, US Department of the Army: *United Textbook of Military Medicine Part 1—Warfare, Weaponry and the Casualty, Medical Aspects of Chemical and Biological Warfare.* Washington, DC, 1997.

[14]The Anthrax: Biological/Toxin Warfare FAQ page. Available at *http://www.geocities.com/area51/station/8320/anthrax.html.*

[15]United States Army Medical Research Institute of Infectious Diseases: *Medical Management of Biological Casualties Handbook* ed 2. Ft. Detrick, Fredrick, MD, 1996.

[16]Ibid, p 31.

[17]US Department of Justice, Federal Emergency Management Agency: *Emergency Response to Terrorism Basic Concepts 1997.* Washington, DC, 1997, p 4–6.

[18]*Emergency Response to Terrorism Basic Concepts 1997,* p 4–9.

[19]*Emergency Response to Terrorism Basic Concepts 1997,* p 4–8.

Appendix A

[1]Firehouse.com. Fellow EMT Arrested in Indiana Medic Slayings page. Available at: *http://www.firehouse.com/news/2001/4/19_dead.html.* Accessed April 20, 2001.

[2]Breister P: "Man Confesses to Killing Campbellsport Woman." *Fond du Lac Reporter* January 8, 2001.

[3]Walker TM: "Two Memphis Bravest, Sheriff's Deputy Shot to Death." *Associated Press* March 8, 2000.

[4]Conley C: "Paramedics Attacked While Rendering Aid." *The Commercial Appeal* February 16, 2000.

[5]Lee HK: "Shots Taken at Oakland Cop, Medics, They Were on Duty Helping Fatally Wounded Man." *San Francisco Chronicle* December 28, 1999.

[6]Gomez J: "Police Search Teen's House." *The News & Observer* December 17, 1999.

[7]Grumet W: "EMT Shot After Climbing Through Window." *Star-Banner* October 27, 1999.

[8]Levine S: "Routine Call Almost Deadly for Paramedic." *The Washington Post* August 10, 1998.

[9]"Gunman Shoots Firefighters Who Had Stopped Traffic." *The Sun* May 4, 1998.

[10]Day J: "Firefighter Felt He Was Going to Die." *The Blade* February 15, 1998.

[11]Gun Left in Greenhouse Slays Perry, Florida Fire Fighter. *International Fire Fighter* 1997; 80/4.

[12]Zekan K: "Moapa Fire Chief Injured in Scuffle." *Las Vegas SUN* October 22, 1997.

[13]"Ambulance Ambushed by Gunfire in Brooklyn." *New York Daily News* February 23, 1997.

[14]DC Fire Fighter Shot While Aiding Shooting Victim in Ambulance. *International Fire Fighter* 1996;79/5:5.

[15]Firehouse.com. Workplace Violence—The Landmine We All Fear page. Available at *http://www.firehouse.com/lodd/2000/memphis/carter.html*. Accessed March 8, 2000.

[16]Fernandez R: "Feigning Injury, Man with Knife Attacks Two Philadelphia Paramedics." *Philadelphia Inquirer* December 26, 1994.

[17]Dunleavy B: Firefighters Fight Fires, Not People. *Firehouse Magazine* 1993;18/8:7.

[18]Denver Fire Fighter Shot and Killed. *International Fire Fighter* 1993;75/1:1.

[19]Fire Fighter Faces Long Recovery After Shooting During LA Riots. *International Fire Fighter* 1992;75/4:10.

Appendix B

[1]Weslager J: Paramedic assault. *Emergency* 1983;15(15):13.

[2]Safariland Ballistics Industries: *Gall's holiday gift catalog* (advertisement). 1988;C3:30.

[3]A 40-page catalog devoted to "the world's best SWAT and hostage rescue team clothing and equipment," now includes emergency medical bags and a med-bag accessory pouch. Brigade Quartermaster: Tactical Catalog 17. Brigade Quartermaster, 1988/1989.

[4]EI Du Pont De Nemours & Co, Industrial Fibers Division, Textile Fibers Department: *Dress for survival, Kevlar personal body armor facts book*, ed 3, Wilmington, DE, EI Du Pont De Nemours & Co, 1987, p 2.

[5]FBI statistics indicate that the percentage of police officers killed with .357 Magnum and 9 mm handguns rose from 13% in 1974 to 35% in 1984. Ibid, p 4.

[6]Ibid, p 3.

Index

Abrasion collar, 128–129

Accident scene, evidence preservation at, 130

Active shooter, 123–124

Aircraft, using
in civil disturbances, 164
TEMS plan for, 113

Ammunition. *See* Bullets

Anhydrous ammonia, 100

Anthrax, 179–180, *181*

Apartment buildings/townhouses
approaching, 37
positioning at, 42

Armed encounter, 22–23
backing away, vehicle, 28–30
calling for assistance in, 30–31
interacting with patient in, 23–26
partner down in, 27–28
survival tips for, 31
vitals pad as distraction in, 26–27

Armor. *See* Soft body armor

Asian gangs, 139–140, 144

Asphyxia, positional, 166–167, 169–170

Assistance calls. *See* Dispatch information

Aum Shinrikyo, 174–175, 179

Automobile. *See entries under* Motor vehicle

Backing away
from domestic encounter, 52–53
from motor vehicle scene, 28–30

Ballistic protection of body armor, 194

Ballistics, 128–129. See also Wound ballistics

Barriers, use in domestic encounters, 51

Barroom situations, 54–58
contact and cover in, 56
crowd control technique in, 57
entering, 55–56
retreating from, 56–57
sizing up, 54–55
survival tips for, 58

Baton rounds/shells, 154–156

Bean bag rounds, 154, 156

Bear hug, breaking away from a, 106–107

Behavior continuum model of hostages, *69*

Binding material, at crime scene, 132

Biologic agents/weapons, 172, 173–174, 178–180
anthrax, 180, *181*
botulinus toxins, *180, 183–184*
cholera, *181, 184*
examples and impact of use of, 178–180
plague, 179, *181–182, 184,* 185
Q fever, *182,* 185
ricin, *184,* 185
smallpox, 179, *182,* 185–186
staphylococcal enterotoxin B, *183–184,* 186
trichothecene mycotoxins, *184,* 186
tularemia, *181–182,* 187
Venezuelan equine encephalitis, *183,* 187
viral hemorrhagic fevers, *183,* 187

Bishops (gang), *142*

Black Disciples (gang), *142*

Black Gangster Disciples, 137, *142,* 143

Blasting caps, 74–75

Blister agents, *176–177,* 178

Blood agents, *176–177,* 178

Bloods (gang), 137, *142*

Boards, as weapons, 81, 82

Body armor. *See* Soft body armor

Body language, in domestic encounters, 49–50

Body position, cover and, 62

Bombs. *See* Explosive devices

Booby traps, 80–82
in drug laboratories, 93–94
at mass-casualty shooting sites, 122
survival tips regarding, 89

Botulinus toxins, 179, 180, *183–184*

Bubonic plague, *181,* 185

Bulletproof vests. *See* Soft body armor

Bullets
cover and concealment from,
60–62
emergency unit protection, 8
rubber, 154–155
wound ballistics, 128–129, 131
Burns, in gang ritual, 140
Buttons (psychological), 50

Cameras, instant, 127
Capture, of hostages, 82–84
Cat's claw, 83–84
Caution, use of, 4–5
at highway incidents, 6–7
at residential incidents, 32–33
Chemical agents/weapons, 172–176
booby traps, 81, 94
explosive, in drug lab, 93–94,
96–97
military agents, 176–178
sarin attack, 174–175
survival tips regarding, 156
tear gas, 149–151
See also Illegal drugs
Chlorine, 177
Chloroacetophenone (CN), 150–151
Choke hold, defending against, 106
Choking agents, *176–177,* 178
Cholera, *181,* 184
Civil disturbances, 157–165
EMS unit tactics in, 164–165
general tactics in, 162–164
preincident planning for, 158–161
riot control agents for, *177,* 178
strategy used in, 161–162
survival tips for, 165
Clostridium botulinum, 180
Clothing
body armor, 2, 159–160
concealment and, 63
evidence preservation and,
129–130
gang-related, 135–137, 141,
142–143, 144–145, 147
protective, fire-related, 95–96
of sexual assault victim, 130
of suspect(s), at mass-casualty
shootings, 124
See also Soft body armor
Club drugs, 97–99
Codes, gang-related, 135
Cold method of methamphetamine
production, 92–93
Cold zone, at contaminated site, 96

Command
briefings, at civil disturbances,
162–163
at mass-casualty shooting site,
121–122
patient restraint and, 168
Command center, in civil disturbances, 160
Communication(s)
at crime scene, documenting,
131–132
with dispatcher. *See* Dispatch information
in domestic encounters, 47–50
force continuum and, 148–149
in mass-casualty shootings,
120–121
with methamphetamine user, 97
restricted, in TEMS planning, 114
in situation requiring force, 102
Concealment
cover and, 59–63
survival tips for, 63
of weapons in motor vehicle,
14–16
Contact and cover
in barroom situation, 56
in gang areas, 145
Contact wounds, 128–129
Coordination of services, 109–110
in civil disturbances, 158
at drug laboratory scene, 95
at mass-casualty shooting scene,
121–122, 124
in preincident training, 124
Corporate gangs, 136
Counseling
in domestic encounters, 53
following hostage experience, 71
Counter Narcotics Terrorism
Operations Medical Support
(CONTOMS) program, 112
Court cases
crime scene evidence in, 130–132
involving patient restraint, 167–168
Cover
in barroom situation, 56
concealment and, 59–63
in gang areas, 145
survival tips for, 63
Coxiella burnetii, 185
"Crank" (drug) production, 90, 91–93
Crazies, hostage-takers as, 66
Crickett (explosive device), *89*

Crime scene, 126–128. See also
    Evidence preservation
Criminals, hostage-takers as, 66
Crips, (gang)137, *142*
Crusaders, hostage-takers as, 66
Crying wolf, 7
Cyanides, 176, *177, 178*
Cyberterrorism, 172

Date-rape drugs, 99–100
Detonating cords, 75
Dispatch information
    in armed encounters, 30–31
    in barroom situations, 58
    difficulties with, 121
    in domestic encounters, 52
    in motor vehicle incidents, 28,
        30–31
    in residential incidents, 33
Distilled mustard agents, 176
Distraction techniques
    in domestic encounters, 51
    at motor vehicle scene, 26–27
    self-defense tactic, 103–104
Documentation
    of assault, 108
    of civil disturbance response plan,
        161
    of crime scene, 130–132
    of patient restraint, 170
    of patient transport, 58
    of TEMS plan, 112–116
Domestic encounters, 46–47
    avoiding violence in, 52–53
    body language in, 49–50
    buttons triggered in, 50
    distraction techniques in, 51
    eye contact in, 49
    separating individuals in, 51
    survival tips for, 53
    voice control in, 47–48
Doors
    at crime scene, 127
    entry and, 41–42, 45
    in hostage situations, 71
Drive-by shootings, 145–146
Driver-side approach to motor vehi-
        cles, 11–15
    to vans, 17–19
Driveways, in residential approach,
    37
Drugs. *See* Illegal drug laboratories;
    Illegal drugs

Ecstasy (drug), 98
El Rukns (gang), 138, *142*
Element of surprise, 4
    in residential approach, 36–37
Elevator, use in residential incident, 42
EME (gang), 138
Emergency care. *See* Patient treatment
Entry
    in barroom situation, 55–56
    at crime scene, 127
    in residential incidents, 41–43
    tier system of, 50–51
Environmental hazards
    at drug laboratory, 96
    TEMS planning and, 114
Equipment. *See* Emergency equip-
        ment; *specific type of equipment*
Escalation of incident, residential sce-
        nario, 33–35
Evidence preservation, 125–132
    approaching crime scene and, 127
    on clothing, 129–130
    critical issues at crime scenes,
        126–128
    documentation and, 130–132
    in sexual assaults, 130
    survival tips for, 132
    types of evidence, 125–127
    wound ballistics, 128–129
Explosive devices, 72–76
    arriving at scene of, 77–78
    booby traps, 80–82, 93–94
    classifications and types of, 74–76
    high/military grade, 172
    makeshift weapons, 82–89
    at mass-casualty shooting sites,
        122
    postexplosion operations, 80
    searching and staging for, 79–80
    survival tips regarding, 89
    training for response to, 76–77
    users of, 73–74

Face-down patient restraint, 167, 169
Females
    date-rape drugs and, 99
    as gang members, 143
    as sexual assault victims, 130
Fighting parties. *See* Barroom situa-
        tions; Domestic encounters
Flak jackets/vests, 159–160
Flash bang devices, 153, 155
Flashlights, in motor vehicle
        approach, 21

Flunitrazepam, 99
Folk Nation (gang), 137–138, 140,
    142, 143
Footwear, gang-related, *142,* 147
Force, reasonable use of, 101–103
Fringe gang members, 136
Front door, positioning at, 41–42

Gamma-butyrolactone (GBL), 99
Gamma-hydroxybutyrate (GHB), 99
Gangs, 133–147
    female members, 143
    graffiti by, 144
    joining, reasons for, 134
    membership levels in, 136–137
    nature of, 134–135
    specific affiliations, *142–143,* 144
        Asian gangs, 139–140
        Hispanic gangs, 138–139
        Midwest gangs, 137–138
        motorcycle gangs, 140–141
        west coast gangs, 137
        white supremacist groups, 141,
            143
    structure and types of, 135–136
    survival tips regarding, 147
    terminology of, 146–147
    territories, working in, 145–146
Gas cylinders, at drug laboratory, 100
Gas shutoff, at drug laboratory,
    96–97
Global Positioning System (GPS), in
    TEMS planning, 113
Graffiti, 138, 144–145
Grenades, 81–82
Guns
    firing effects of, 128
    handmade, *88*
    See also Bullets; Wound ballistics
Gunshot wounds, 128–129

Hair, from crime scene, 126
Hand signs, gang-related, 135–136,
    137, 138, 147
Hand washing, at crime scene, 132
Handgrenades, 81–82
Hard contact wounds, 128–129
Hardcore gang members, 136
Hazardous materials response team, at
    drug laboratory, 94–95, 96
Hazards, TEMS planning and, 114
Headlock, breaking, 104
Head-on approach to motor vehicle,
    19

Helicopter. *See* Aircraft, using
Hell's Angels (motorcycle gang), 140
Highway incidents, 6–9
    indicating need for caution, 6–7
    positioning unit during, 7–8
    preparing to leave unit during, 8–9
    survival tips for, 9
    See also Motor vehicles, approach-
        ing
Hispanic gangs, 138–139
Hog-tying, 167, 169–170
Hospitals, TEMS planning and, 114
Hostage situations, 64–71
    holding of, *67,* 68–70
    hostage-takers, 66
    law enforcement procedures in,
        70–71
    stages of, 66–70
    Stockholm Syndrome in, 70
    surviving, 65, 71
Hot zone, at contaminated site,
    94–97
Hypoxia, 167

Identifiers, of gangs, *142–143*
Illegal drug laboratories, 90–100
    agencies responding to, 95
    emergency scene operations at,
        94–95
    encountering, 95
    fire suppression operations at,
        95–96
    hazards of, 93–94
    location of, 91
    methamphetamine, equipment in,
        92
    monitoring emergency personnel
        at, 97
    positive-pressure ventilation at,
        96–97
    recognizing, 91–93
    sales by and proliferation of, 90–91
    survival tips regarding, 100
Illegal drugs, 90
    club drugs, 97–99
    methamphetamine, 90, 91–92, 97
Insignia, gang-related, 137–139, *141,*
    144–145
Intermediate-range wounds, 129
Interview stance, 103
Irritants, *177,* 178

Jails. *See* Prisons
Jump kit, 11, 12, 16, 19

Ketamine (K), 99
Key ring, as weapon, 83, 87
Kill zone
    of motor vehicles, 15, 16, 18
    of residence, 42, 43
Knocked down, defensive response,
    107
Ku Klux Klan, 141

La Nuestra Familia (gang), 138
Landing zone (LZ), TEMS planning
    and, 113
Latin Disciples (gang), 142
Latin Kings (gang), 137, 142, 144
Law enforcement
    civil disturbances, predicting, 158
    explosive devices and, 79–80
    hostage situation procedures,
        70–71
Less-lethal munitions, 148–156
    force continuum, 148–149
    light/sound diversionary devices,
        153
    OC spray, 151–152
    projectiles, 154–156
    survival tips regarding, 156
    Tasers, 153–154
    tear gas, 149–151
Lewisite (L), 176–177
Light/sound diversionary devices,
    153
Litigation. See Court cases
LNF (gang), 138
Location
    of illegal drug laboratories, 91
    of staging area in civil disturbances,
        160
Low explosives, 74
Lysergic acid diethylamide (LSD),
    98–99

Makeshift weapons, 82–89
Maps, in TEMS planning, 113–114
Mara Salvatrucha (MS) (gang),
    138–139, 143
Mass-casualty shootings, 117–124
    communication in, 120–121
    incidents of, 118–119
    preincident planning for, 117, 120
    site command at, 121–122
    site operations at, 122–124
    survival tips for, 124
Media, at mass-casualty shootings,
    124

Methamphetamine production,
    90–93
Methamphetamine user, interacting
    with, 97
3,4-Methylenedioxymethamphetamine
    (MDMA), 98
Mexican Mafia (gang), 138
Midwest gangs, 137–138
Military chemical agents, 176–178
Motor vehicle accidents, evidence
    preservation at, 130
Motor vehicles
    columns in, 13, 18
    concealing weapons in, 14
Motor vehicles, approaching,
    10–21
    armed patient and. See Armed
        encounter
    driver-side approach, 11–15
    head-on approach, 19
    passenger-side approach, 15–17
    patient treatment and, 20
    survival tips for, 20–21
    vans, 17–19
    See also Highway incidents
Motorcycle gangs, 140–141, 147
Moving, of hostages, 67
Munitions. See Weapons
Mustard agents, 176
Mutual aid, in civil disturbances,
    160

Near contact wounds, 129
Nerve agents, 176, 178
Nuclear terrorism, 172

Oleoresin capsicum (OC) spray,
    150–152
Orto-chlorobenzylidene-malononitrile
    (CS), 150–151
Outlaw motorcycle gangs (OMG),
    140–141

Package bomb indicators, 79
Partner down, at motor vehicle scene,
    27–28
Passengers of motor vehicle
    in driver-side approach, 13–14
    exit of, response to, 21
    in passenger-side approach,
        15–17
Passenger-side approach to motor
    vehicles, 15–17
    to vans, 17–18

Patient
   armed. *See* Armed encounter
   as crime victim. *See* Evidence
      preservation
   statement by, documenting, 131
   treatment. *See* Patient treatment
Patient restraint, 166–170
   armed patient, 24, 31
   court cases over, 167–168
   criteria for, 168
   procedures/techniques of, 167–169
   survival tips for, 170
Patient treatment
   in armed encounter, 23–24
   in barroom situation, 56–57
   biologic/chemical weapon victims.
      See specific agent
   at crime scene, 127–129
   at drive-by shooting, 145–146
   force continuum and, 148–149
   at motor vehicle scene, 20
   OC spray victim, 152
   sexual assault victim, 100, 130
   Taser victim, 153–154
   tear gas victim, 150–151
Patrol car. *See* Emergency response
   unit
Pedestrian accident, evidence preser-
   vation at, 130
People Nation (gang), 137–138, *142,*
   143
Phosgene oxime (CX), *176–177*
Photography, at crime scene, 127
Phrases to avoid, *47*
Physical evidence, 125–126. See also
   Evidence preservation
Plague, *181–182, 184–185*
Planning. *See* Preincident planning
Pneumonic plague, *181,* 185
Police officer, being mistaken for,
   3–4
Politics, gangs in, 135
Positive-pressure ventilation, 96–97
Positional asphyxia, 166–167,
   169–170
Powder burns, 129
Pre-fire planning, 120
Preincident planning
   for civil disturbances, 158–161
   for mass-casualty shootings, 117,
      120
   by TEMS team, 112–116
   See also Training

Preservation of evidence. *See* Evidence
   preservation
Primary high explosives, 74–76
Prisons
   gangs in, 135, 138
   restraint teams in, 168
Professionalism, in domestic encoun-
   ters, 48
Projectile weapons, 154–156
Prone position, in patient restraint,
   167, 170
Protective clothing, fire-related, 95–96
Pulmonary agents, *176–177,* 178

Q fever, *182,* 185

Racism, white supremacists and, 141,
   143
Radiologic terrorism, 172
Radios
   800-MHz system, 121
Rear bear hug, breaking away from,
   106–107
Relief personnel, 160
Reputation, gangs and, 137
Residential incidents, 32–39
   approaching, 37–39
   arriving at, 35–37
   escalation scenario, 33–35
   moving into/through structure, 42–44
   positioning at front door, 41–42
   survival tips for, 39, 45
   weapons in, 44–45
   See also Domestic encounters
Resolution, of hostage situation, 67
Resource identification, in TEMS plan-
   ning, 115
Respect
   in domestic encounters, 48
   gangs and, 137
Restraint. *See* Patient restraint
Retaliation, gangs and, 137
Retreat
   from barroom situation, 56–57
   from fires in civil disturbances, 164
Ricin, *184,* 185
Riot control agents, 167, *177,* 178
Riots. *See* Civil disturbances
Rohypnol, 99
Rubber bullets/batons, 154–156

Sarin attack, 174–175
Scars, of gang members, 140
Scavenger gangs, 136

School incidents. *See* Mass-casualty
shootings
Search for weapons/explosive devices,
79–80, 83–84
Secondary high explosives, 74–76
Self-defense tactics, 101–108
breaking holds, 103–107
distracting assailant, 103–104
documenting, 108
from ground, 107
interview stance, 103
practicing, 107–108
survival tips, 108
tweaking assailant, 104
using reasonable force with, 101–103
See also Less-lethal weapons
Self-protection, 1–2, 4–5
Sexual assaults, evidence preservation
in, 100, 130
Shootings
active shooter, 123–124
drive-by, 145–146
See also Bullets; Mass-casualty
shootings; Wound ballistics
Sirens. *See* Warning lights and sirens
Site visit, in TEMS planning, 113
Skin, bullet wounds, 128–129
Skinheads, 141, 143
Smallpox, *182,* 185–186
Soft body armor, 192–194
ballistic protection from, 194
characteristics and care of, 192–193
identifying sources of, 159
Soot, in hard contact wounds, 129
Soreños (gang), 138, *143*
Special Weapons and Tactics (SWAT)
teams
at mass-casualty shooting sites,
123–124
tactical medics and, 108–112
"Speed" (drug) production, 90, 91–93
Staging areas, in civil disturbances, 160
Staphylococcal enterotoxin B (SEB),
183–184, 186
Star-shaped bullet wounds, 129
Statements at crime scene, document-
ing, 131
Stingball Grenade, 155
Stockholm Syndrome, 70
Stranglehold, breaking away from a
in attack from above, 107
in frontal attack, 104
in rear attack, 105–106
Structure, entering. *See* Entry

Suicide attempt
responding to, 39
"Suicide by cop," 149
Surprise, element of, 4
Surveillance, of hostages, 67
Survival tips
armed encounter, 31
barroom situations, 58
civil disturbances, 165
cover and concealment, 63
domestic encounters, 53
drug laboratories, 100
entering a structure, 45
evidence preservation, 132
explosive devices, 89
gangs, 147
highway incidents, 9
hostage situations, 71
less lethal weapons, 156
mass-casualty shootings, 124
motor vehicle approach, 20–21
patient restraint, 170
residential incidents, 39
self-defense tactics, 108
TEMS, 116
threat and need, 5
SWAT medics. *See* Tactical Emergency
Medical Support

Tactical Emergency Medical Support
(TEMS), 109–116
mission planning by, 112–116
program goals of, 111–112
survival tips regarding, 116
SWAT teams and, 110
training program for, 112
Tags, gang-related, 144
Talkgroups, 121
Tasers, 153–154
Task force operations in civil disturbances, 161–165
Tattoos, gang-related, 138, 141
Tear gas, 149–150
Terminology
gang-related, 146–147
phrases to avoid, 47
Territorial gangs, 136
Terrorism, 171–188
biologic, 178–187
chemical, 174–178
defined, 172
overview, 171–174
Testimonial evidence
defined, 125–126

Testimonial evidence (*Continued*)
    providing, in court case, 130–132
    See also Evidence preservation
Threat of violence, preparation for
    facing, 1–2, 5
Tier entry system, in domestic
    encounters, 50–51
Tiny Rascals Gang, 140, *143*, 144
Towels, at crime scene, 132
Townhouses. *See* Apartment build-
    ings/townhouses
Trace evidence, 126–127
Training
    for handling explosive devices, 76
    NFPA 1500 requirement for, 5
    preincident joint efforts, 124
    revised approach to, 4
    in TEMS program, 112, 116
Transport
    of hostages, 67–68
    of OC spray victim, 152
    of Taser victim, 153–154
Traumatic suicide, 39
Treatment of patient. *See* Patient
    treatment
Trichothecene mycotoxins (T2), *184,*
    186
Trunk lid, in motor vehicle approach,
    12–13, 16
Tularemia, *181–182,* 187
Tweak, as self-defense tactic, 104

Urine samples, of sexual assault
    victim, 100
US government, terrorism expendi-
    tures, 172–173

Vans, approaching, 17–19
Variola virus, 185–186
Vehicle. *See* Emergency response unit;
    entries under Motor vehicle
Venezuelan equine encephalitis, *183,*
    187
Ventilation
    positive-pressure, 96–97
Vesicant agents, *176–177,* 178
Vice Lords (gang), 137, *142,* 143
Violence, preparing for threat of, 1–2
Viral hemorrhagic fevers, (VHF) *183,*
    187
Vital signs, of restrained patient, 170
Vitals pad, distracting armed patient
    with, 26–27
Voice control, in domestic encounters,
    47–48

Walls, as cover, 61–62
Wannabee gang members, 137
Warm zone, at contaminated site,
    95–96
Warning lights and sirens, 35–36
Weapons
    of armed patient, 23–26, 31
    biologic. *See* Biologic
        agents/weapons
    bombs. *See* Explosive devices
    chemical. *See* Chemical
        agents/weapons
    concealment in motor vehicle,
        13–17, 21
    discharge by vehicular passenger,
        22–23
    force continuum, 148–149
    of gang members, 141, 147
    light/sound diversionary devices,
        153
    makeshift, 82–89
    OC spray, 151–152
    projectile weapons, 154–156
    in residence, 44–45
    searching patients for, 83–84
    for self-protection, 2
    survival tips regarding, 5, 89
    Tasers, 153–154
    tear gas, 149–151
    TEMS and, 112
    in vans, 17
    wound ballistics, 128–129, 154,
        155, 156
"Weapons of mass destruction"
    (WMD), 172
"Weapons of mass effect" (WME),
    172
Weather, TEMS planning and,
    114–115
West coast gangs, 137
White supremacist groups, 141,
    143
Windows
    entry, 45
    in hostage situations, 71
    shatter proofing, 165
Women. *See* Females
Wound ballistics
    documenting, 131
    from less-lethal weapons,
        154–156
    from lethal weapons, 128–129
Wrist grasp, 103

Zones, of contaminated site, 94–97